REBOOTING

MY

BRAIN

REBOOTING

MY

BRAIN

How A Freak Aneurysm Reframed My Life

BY **Maria Ross**

Cover design and print layout: Juli Saeger Russell

Author photo: Alison Jensen, www.alisonjensen.com

Library of Congress Control Number: 2011961696
ISBN: 978-0-9848939-0-4

ATTENTION CORPORATIONS, UNIVERSITIES, COLLEGES AND
PROFESSIONAL ORGANIZATIONS:

Quantity discounts are available on bulk purchases of this book for educational, gift purposes, or as premium items. Special books or book excerpts can also be created to fit specific needs. For information, please contact Red Slice Press at info@red-slice.com

A NOTE TO MY READERS

My MISSION WITH this book is twofold: to share what I hope you find an inspirational story of triumph over adversity, and to reveal some of what I've learned about brain injuries. I hope I can inspire others through the lessons I learned so that they can pick themselves up and dust themselves off after life knocks the wind right out of them. It is also my intent to provide a patient perspective on just how tough it can be to deal with a severe brain injury. Perhaps this will help make things easier for other brain injury survivors and their families, as well as provide some resources I found helpful in my situation. It is important they know they are not alone in regards to many personality, emotional or cognitive changes they may have experienced.

As you read my tale, please remember this is a memoir about my own personal experiences, interpretations and impressions. It is not meant to be a medical journal, scientific book or diagnostic tool. While I have made every attempt to provide accurate information and have cited sources where appropriate, **please understand that neither I nor this book are dispensing medical advice, and I do not intend any of this information to be used for self-diagnosis or treatment.** This is merely a chronicle of my own personal journey. Other people's particular needs, experiences and recovery processes may differ. If you have any questions or concerns about your health, including headaches, health risks and post-brain-injury recovery, you should contact your own physician or healthcare provider.

I hope you enjoy my story. I would be honored if you'd share it with anyone you know facing brain-injury challenges, particularly those impacted personally or through their friends and family. The more we can educate ourselves and others about the surprising and often unseen effects of brain injury, the more healing and understanding there will be for patients and their families.

This book is dedicated to the millions of people each year who suffer from both traumatic and acquired brain injuries that impact their bodies, livelihoods and personal lives. You are not alone.

Best,

Maria Ross

CONTENTS

(CONTINUED)

PROLOGUE

August 2008
Seattle, Washington

I woke up when someone wheeled my bed—with me in it—from my hospital room. Even before I opened my eyes, I knew something wasn't right. After opening them, I could see only blurry shapes and faint outlines of color, as if I were looking through a dirty glass.

My brain, which I didn't yet know was damaged, tried to fill in what was happening. I decided the nurses were moving all the patients into the hallway, lining us up head-to-toe along the upper-floor railing. Their shoes shuffled along the faux marble floors and voices whispered urgently in the darkness.

What the heck was going on? Why were they sneaking us all out into the hall in the middle of the night?

Sobbing, I begged a nurse to call my husband. She shook her head no. She was probably trying to hide her evil deeds, I thought. I felt for the phone and miraculously punched in my home phone number, just by touch. How on earth did I remember it when I couldn't remember which city I lived in? On the other end, Paul mumbled as he fought his way back to wakefulness. It was three a.m.

"Come get me, honey!" I covered the phone and tried to keep my sobbing voice low. "They've put us all in the hallway. *What are they doing to us?*"

He tried to soothe me. At some point he did calm me down, and the nurse returned the receiver to the cradle. I drifted back to sleep.

Paul, on the other hand, lay wide awake. His lively, intelligent wife now sounded like the paranoid conspiracy theorists she used to mock on their favorite TV crime dramas. What do you do when your spouse becomes a different person, literally overnight?

Later, I learned my mind had tricked me. While I imagined I was trapped in an endless corridor, I had actually been wheeled to a private room. The nurse had tried to explain this, to no avail. Relenting at last, she was the one—not me—who had dialed my husband, thinking he might be the only person to assuage my fears. There had been no sinister plot, no patient abuse. It was simply my damaged brain, playing one of the many tricks it would play on me as it tried to repair itself from the recent trauma.

Unfortunately, Paul received similar panicked, but unfounded, phone calls over the next several nights, not just one.

The neurosurgeons had warned Paul after I was rushed unconscious to the emergency room, "We can save her life, Mr. Ross, but that's all we can do. We have no idea yet what effect this hemorrhage had on her brain, memories, motor skills or personality."

We spent the next year and beyond learning what those effects would be.

PART ONE

Life As We Knew It

You may not realize it when it happens, but a kick in the teeth may be the best thing in the world for you.

- Walt Disney

There's nothing that cleanses your soul like getting the hell kicked out of you.

- Woody Hayes

THE STORM BEFORE THE STORM

İT ALL STARTED with a theatre audition.

Actually, I have to go further back than that. It started with the idea to move to Seattle in 2007. Loving the San Francisco Bay area but unable to afford a house without having to pour every spare dollar into a mortgage, Paul and I decided to transplant our newly married selves up to the Pacific Northwest.

It was a crazy year. Paul had just secured his Green Card, which meant my new Scottish husband was no longer beholden to his company for a work visa. A few years earlier, unafraid and looking for a change, he had transferred from Oxford, England, to San Francisco to work at our software company's corporate headquarters. We met. We became friends. And then we fell in love. Many thought our coupling an odd one: me, the extroverted, energetic and optimistic straight-A student who loves being on stage and competing in bar trivia contests, and Paul, the introverted, wry, often curmudgeonly Scotsman who prefers small group get-togethers over big bashes, and who loves video games and cycling alone in the Marin hills. I fell in love with his wide green eyes set behind sleek wireframe glasses, his dimple and his witty banter. Our relationship was easy from the start; we were just as content kicking back on the couch to watch an indie film as we were hitting the bars with friends to celebrate a birthday…or a Tuesday.

After calling off an engagement with my college sweetheart, throwing myself into—and out of—a toxic relationship and laughing through a few more years of crazy dating sagas, I joyfully cried, "Yes!" when this well-adjusted man who adored me proposed on a hike in a redwood grove. I was thirty-two. I knew he was the guy for me and it was time.

Ever the achiever, I was always looking for the next step up at work—
without thinking about whether I really wanted it or not. On fast tracks,
we both got promoted in different areas of marketing for our multinational
software company and happily planned our wedding while riding a double
wave of career success and good fortune. The money was great and enabled
us to pay off all of our debts. When I say "our," I really mean "my" credit
card bills from years spent skiing in Tahoe, drinking wine in Napa and
eating out at San Francisco's amazing restaurants. In sharp contrast, Paul
had come over from the UK with his suitcase, his bikes and a laptop, and
he had invested only in the bare necessities upon getting settled. We quickly
began stashing away money for our first house.

Swinging to the next big job opportunity, I was recruited away to be
a director of corporate marketing at a small technology company, which
meant jumping back into a small-company environment for more control
and impact. I was psyched. I worked with a team I loved and we were on
fire. There was so much to do and scant resources to get it done. We made
great strides but the days blurred together in a whirlwind of stress and
activity. The to-do list never shrank and our Marketing team's initial shiny,
happy reception was now met with even more demands. That's the curse of
competence, I guess: the more you do really well, the more people expect.

While I adored my team, I hated the daily budget fights we had with the
CFO, the fights for respect from the sales team and the fights for the CEO
to trust our expertise and follow our advice to help the company grow.
Some days, I felt like it was our small but mighty marketing team against
the world. As Paul began his job search post-Green Card, we talked about
leaving San Francisco and starting fresh somewhere else.

Chicago was briefly considered, as I had once lived there and loved the
urban life in the Windy City with its amazing restaurants and museums.
It was also closer to my family in the Midwest. But we both couldn't
imagine going back to bone-chilling winters and scraping snow off the car
every morning after having lived for years on the mild West Coast. Seattle,
Washington, and Portland, Oregon, became strong alternates to the Bay
Area—and both were more affordable to boot.

"Why don't you just work with recruiters in the Bay Area and Seattle
and we'll let the job opportunity decide where we go?" I suggested.
He agreed.

Seattle-based Microsoft soon came calling, as did some small up-and-
coming Bay Area companies. Paul had his pick. Weighing the options, we

looked at everything Microsoft offered—experience, opportunity and killer benefits.

Those benefits would later save our peace of mind and bank account in ways we couldn't possibly imagine at the time.

With Paul's job acceptance, we headed north. I kept my job and worked remotely from home, since I managed all my contractors over email and phone anyway. In my spare time, I researched hanging out my own shingle and becoming a freelance marketing consultant. This arrangement actually became the perfect transition.

What a whirlwind.

Paul had to start his job in Seattle in August, two months before I could join him. Besides being a marketer, I am also an actress on the side and active in the theatre scene. At that time, I was in a play—a comedic satire of *Citizen Kane*—and our performances lasted into October. I wanted to see it through.

In August, I juggled the frustrating tech job, the play rehearsals—and buying a house. Paul and I went up to Seattle to house hunt and after seeing over ten houses in two days, we decided to place an offer on a fabulous new townhome in Seattle's Queen Anne neighborhood. We did all the paperwork via Fed Ex since we were in two different places. But we got through our first house-buying and mortgage experience relatively quickly and unscathed.

Settled in by October 2007, just in time to celebrate my thirty-fifth birthday, we began our new life. We already had some great friends in Seattle—Barb and Guy—but they were the only ones we knew. Guy had worked with both of us at our previous company. Lanky and tall, he's got the most laughing blue eyes I've ever seen and he's quick with a huge smile, hug or enthusiastic cheer of support. He's always game to do something fun and, very much like me, gets excited by the idea of a weekend trip to Mexico or renting a ski chalet in France without thinking through the logistics. Barb, a brunette beauty with warm, intelligent eyes and an easy smile, is his counterpoint: practical, analytical and able to take a step back to think things through. We often joke that Barb is Paul and Guy is me in our respective marriages. Barb and Paul are the calming influences against our whirling dervish personalities. Thank God that Guy and I can orbit around people like that and each couple can create a harmonious duo greater than the sum of its parts.

Barb and Guy introduced us to their circle and I also contacted folks with whom friends had set me up. It felt like online dating. I typically emailed someone I had never met after our mutual friend made an introduction, and met them in a bar or coffee shop somewhere, not quite knowing what to expect.

Many afternoons found me clutching my latte at a table alone, fretting, "Does my hair look okay? Is that person who just walked through the door the person I'm supposed to meet? Act casual! Do people think I'm being stood up?"

Some folks I clicked with, others I did not. I slowly expanded my small network.

January 2008 came along and we started looking for a dog. Both Paul and I grew up with dogs and knew we wanted one. Soon Eddie, a skittish and petite (forty pounds fully grown) Black Lab mix with soulful eyes and a bouncy step joined our family after just one visit to the animal shelter. Thank God he was already housetrained, but we went the rounds of obedience training, struggling with taking control of "the walk" and acclimating to caring and feeding another little creature. It was like getting used to a new baby, but with less screaming and more sleep.

It was around this time that my company finally decided to lay off staff in order to trim costs. Thankfully, I'd been mentally gearing up the consulting practice and was told about the layoff one morning, which I already knew was coming and had secretly hoped for so I'd have no excuse not to try my hand at entrepreneurship. By that same afternoon, my website went live and I notified my entire network that Red Slice, my branding and marketing consultancy, was open for business. I eagerly started networking, consulting with lawyers and accountants, and learning how to be a business owner.

So let's review: New job for Paul, new city for us, new house, new dog, new business, new friends, new routine, new favorite hangouts, and new life. Talk about a perfect storm of extreme stress. Absorbing all of this change sucked the energy right out of us. Most nights, we fell into bed, exhausted.

Oh, and lest I forget: I was also learning all about the Seattle acting scene and investigating audition opportunities. Life was a frenzy but it was going to be great, we said. With my own freelance business, I was going to have oodles of time to act and write, my two favorite passions. Ha. When you're running your own business, I once heard someone say, you can work whenever you want. As long as its twenty-four hours a day, seven days a week.

So now that you have the lay of the land, let's pick up where we left off. It all started with a theatre audition...

Early June, 2008
I trekked out to Issaquah, a lovely little town about fifteen minutes east of Seattle. The Village Theatre was holding open auditions for their entire season and I hoped to get cast in *The Importance of Being Earnest*. I'm a huge fan of comedic period pieces. I drove to the quaint old downtown that seemed frozen in another era and parked near the marquee of the historic theatre. How exciting! A real theatre—not a makeshift industrial space that was the norm for the independent theatre scene I'd been used to back in San Francisco. I rehearsed my two monologues in the lobby, did my vocal exercises, warmed up my tongue, and even did a few side stretches and jumping jacks to loosen up.

"Maria Ross?"

I was up. As I entered the majestic old theatre, it was somewhat dark but the stage was lit like an interrogation room. Heart racing and palms sweating, I said hello to the barely visible four auditors seated in the middle row and confidently marched onto the stage. The great thing about being in this scenario is that you actually can't see their faces very well and for me, that makes it easier to let loose and perform. I can't see if they hate it or not.

I performed my two monologues, probably too fast. But I never let my nerves show. My heart was pounding in my ears but I ignored it. I'd done this enough times to know how to just ignore all the fear and focus on the performance as much as I can.

"Thank you very much, Maria. That was great."

"Well, thank you for the opportunity to audition today." It always helps to be polite and professional so they don't assume you'll be a diva.

I stepped off stage and walked back up the aisle as my nerves "came down." A calm wave washed over my tense muscles as adrenaline subsided and I took a deep, luxurious breath. My pulse slowly returned to normal.

Or so I thought.

When I had almost reached the rear door, I faltered. The blood in my head felt as if it rushed down to my feet like a released grain chute, leaving me lightheaded. Where one second there had been no pain, a huge spike was suddenly pounded into the top of my head, blinding me.

I grabbed for a nearby pole. My neck muscles cramped in stubborn agony and soon my entire back seized up as if I had just lifted too heavy of a weight. Nausea set in as I struggled to comprehend what had happened to me in the last five seconds. Swiftly gulping air in and out, I tried to regulate my breathing, and thought this was just a serious case of performance anxiety.

I walked to the lobby restroom as if a book was balanced on my head, trying hard not to upset a single muscle for fear of collapsing like a house of cards. Mercifully, no one was in there as I fumbled to the sink to splash cold water on my face. Years ago in kindergarten, we'd had a particularly hot spring in New York. My teacher told us we could cool down by running cold water over the inside of our wrists. Not sure why it works, but it does. I heeded her advice in that theatre bathroom and thought, "Wow, you must have been so nervous that your blood pressure spiked. Let's just work on bringing you back down, missy."

High blood pressure runs in my family. Being a Type A personality myself, I have had bouts of it in the past. At one point in my early thirties, I needed medication for the high blood pressure, but then it settled down— perhaps after I finally dumped the toxic boyfriend—and I was able to go off the pills.

Shocked and still disoriented, I thought maybe this was just an extreme reaction to the nerves and stress during the last few months.

Proud that I had avoided passing out or throwing up, I thought I had everything under control. But as I turned away from the sink, my neck and back pain came back into sharp focus and I couldn't turn my head or even stand up straight without tears springing to my eyes. I somehow managed to make my way out to my car.

"Let's just sit for a while and get some fresh air, and you'll be fine," I reassured myself. I sat in the driver's seat and leaned against the headrest with my eyes closed for about twenty minutes. Breathing deeply and fighting back tears of confusion, I focused on simply stabilizing myself enough to drive back to Seattle. Daggers shot up and down my neck if I turned the wrong way, so I moved as if I were in a full body cast to keep the pain at bay. Satisfied I was stabilized, I turned the key and slowly drove away.

Paul was at a dentist appointment downtown, and I was supposed to pick him up on my way home. I couldn't even call him from the road because that would have meant moving my head around too much to deal with the cell phone. Pulling into a parking spot to wait for him, I finally reached the phone and dialed it to let him know I was there.

"Babe, you need to drive when you come down. Something happened and I can't move my back and neck. I'm in so much pain," I told him.

Trotting to the car, he opened the driver side door for me. I eased myself out as carefully as I could and went around to the passenger side.

He looked at me, puzzled. "What happened?"

"I have no idea. One second I was fine and the next I had a blinding migraine. The pain zoomed from zero to sixty in less than three seconds. I can't even move. Let's get home before I get nauseous again."

Paul obliged. We stopped off for migraine medicine to try to deal with things ourselves. I took the pills and crawled into bed.

Paul hugged and kissed me that night before I went to sleep, like he always does. With a furrowed brow, he watched me as I fell asleep. He really wanted me to be happy in Seattle.

And this was not boding well.

THERE ARE HEADACHES . . . AND THEN THERE ARE *HEADACHES*

Headaches like that don't just happen, at least not to me. It was sudden and excruciatingly painful, and it immobilized my neck and back. I'd had mild migraines before but I knew this was no ordinary headache.

I immediately looked for a doctor. We were new in town so we didn't have one lined up yet. Because I'd moved several times in my life, I had a standard "getting settled" checklist for each new city. Finding a new primary-care doctor was definitely on that list, but I had been waiting for my yearly physical to roll around in the fall before dealing with it. This little hitch pushed that search forward.

I found Dr. C through our health care provider website. In his online video, he made earnest eye contact, spoke in layman's terms and focused on his patients' feelings, rather than just their symptoms. I immediately warmed to his empathetic boy-next-door approach. I made an appointment for the next day, saying I had to get in to see him because I was pretty much immobilized.

Dr. C's office was easy to find. A huge waiting room greeted me when I checked in. I had driven myself there; the pain was still severe but manageable. They called me in before I even had a chance to fill out all the paperwork.

"So nice to meet you, Maria. Sounds like you're having some headache issues?" He was kind and I liked the way he actively listened and didn't just usher me through the assembly line.

I told him about the sudden episode, my high blood pressure history and all the stress and change that had been going on in our lives. He took my blood pressure. It was something ridiculous, like 150 over 110.

"Well, it's really high and maybe that is what is causing the migraine," he said. "We could try putting you on blood pressure medication again."

"I'd like to see if I can get it down without medication," I said. "Maybe as I settle into things, into my business, I can try to get it down through yoga or acupuncture?" I was desperate to at least try a natural way first and leave daily pills as a last resort. "Would going off my birth control pill help at all?"

"Maybe, maybe not," he said. "You shouldn't be on them anyway with that blood pressure so high right now." Dr. C took some notes. "Okay, let's try to have you manage this for about a month and see how it impacts your headaches. Watch your sodium intake, get back to yoga, and give acupuncture a try."

Relieved at knowing this might just all be high blood pressure and not something more drastic, I told him I'd need to talk to Paul first about going off birth control, and I would call him to let him know about the plan.

"Here's my direct office line," he said as he handed me a card. "Let's start monitoring your blood pressure nightly and tracking it. Buy one of those home monitors at the drugstore. Call me when you make a decision about the pill or if you have any other questions. And I'm prescribing a few weeks of physical therapy for the neck and back pain, which you can start right away."

I really liked this guy.

"If the blood pressure readings are still high after about a month and the headaches are just as severe and frequent, call me and come back in. We may need to put you on medication at that point."

Off I went. The neck and back pain, while lessened, were still a nuisance so I immediately went to the physical therapy (PT) clinic a few floors below Dr. C's office to make my appointments. The headache had come and gone in the days since the initial event, usually returning in a "slow burn" kind of way. I managed it with ibuprofen and over-the-counter migraine medicine.

My physical therapist and I worked on strengthening exercises, stretches and light massage. As she poked and kneaded, I could indeed feel the muscles relaxing, so I thought we were on our way. After our sessions, my headaches were usually less severe or in some cases completely dissolved.

At the time, I was working on a part-time project at Microsoft (in a different department than where Paul worked) and was only required to drive into the office one or two days a week. The rest of the time, I worked from home, which was ideal. With our dog, Eddie, around, it was nice to have the flexibility to walk him every morning along the tree-lined Fremont Ship Canal before starting my work day.

I loved my new career as a marketing consultant. Before the Microsoft project came along, I had one or two small clients that I got through the amazing Melody Biringer, a sassy Seattle entrepreneur who knows everyone. She and I met through a new business incubator I attended, and we became fast friends. She introduced me around town and helped me land a plum project with another uber-connected woman on a big event. This event, to be held at the top of the posh Columbia Tower Club, was an invitation-only retreat with some of Seattle's most powerful women executives. And here I was, just starting my business with this rare opportunity to build such bridges. It was the dream of a young entrepreneur's life.

The event was held on June 19, a few weeks after the first debilitating headache and subsequent visit with Dr. C. By this time, I still had the headaches off and on, but never as severe as that first one had been.

On the day of the Columbia Tower event, I called Dr. C during a break to ask a few final questions about going off the birth control pill. Paul and I had decided to do whatever was needed to bring my blood pressure down, and Dr. C applauded our decisions. Never before had a doctor spent so much time on the phone answering my questions and calming my nerves.

He also asked how the blood pressure readings were going.

"Well, the readings are lower on the days I have acupuncture or therapy, but even those lower readings are still really high," I admitted.

"Okay. Just keep an eye on it, and call me if that continues after you go off the pill."

The next month or so was filled with working on the Microsoft project, marketing my business and managing my blood pressure. I continued to suffer from the bad headaches every now and then. When my back and neck pain flared up, I couldn't always make it to yoga, so I tried acupuncture for the first time and really liked it. It felt a little weird to lie face down on a table and know the acupuncturist was sticking small needles into my skin but, somehow, it helped the pain. Certainly that could be due to the acupuncture itself and to the alignment of chi flow, chakras and whatnot... or to the fact that you spend about twenty silent and juicy minutes relaxing in a dimly lit room. I'm sure that has something to do with it, too.

Having always eaten reasonably healthy, Paul and I stepped it up by using less salt and reading labels for sodium intake. Good Lord, there is a lot of sodium in what we eat. Pre-packaged soups are the worst culprits, with sometimes about 50 percent of our daily sodium intake in one serving.

Look at me, I thought. What with the regular yoga, the acupuncture treatments and my expanded food consciousness, I've really gone "Pacific Northwest." I'm fitting right in, here in Seattle. Now I just need to go vegan and I'll have all my bases covered.

Unfortunately, the headache came back every so often. On a few occasions, the migraine made me so nauseous that I'd be vomiting once or twice a day. But I powered through, diligently taking my blood pressure readings and trusting the doctor.

Every night, I'd place the cuff on my arm and try to relax. After two readings to get an average, I wrote down all the numbers on a notepad in my bedside drawer. A normal blood pressure reading is about 120 over 80. Above that, and it steps into hypertension. My readings ranged from 140 over 100 to sometimes 160 over 120. I even remember a few readings of 170 over something. These could not possibly be 100 percent accurate, I thought, and I chalked them up to the cheap monitor having less than stellar accuracy.

"What is it tonight?" Paul asked, trying to be nonchalant.

I told him. He stared back at me.

"Dr. C said to give it a month or two," I often reminded my dear husband. And we both went to bed wrapped up in our own worry.

I can't remember which headache and vomiting episode put me over the edge, but I knew it was time to call Dr. C and schedule a return visit.

Actually, that episode must have been during the week prior to August 4, 2008...because I never got the chance to call him, once that fateful day dawned.

On the weekend before August 4, I was delighted that our good friends Scott and Carrie were visiting from Indianapolis. Scott—with his wild curly hair, hearty laugh and devotion to England's Arsenal Football Club—is a creative genius and runs a successful branding firm. An art school graduate, he loathes blind conformity and tolerates my sorority girl exuberance and love for boy bands only because they're genuine. Scott was in town because of some client work at Microsoft. (Yes, everything in my life seems to come back around to Bill Gates.)

Scott's wife, Carrie, had tagged along to see me. Our friendship began while working together at an Indianapolis ad agency in the late 1990s. I'm not quite sure why we kept our distance initially: perhaps I was a little intimidated by her smarts and beauty and maybe she assumed I was a typical, uncreative "suit"—even though at the time she was one as well.

But her talents have always lain in the written word, and she was biding time in an account management position so she could eventually move up to the copywriting floor.

A raven-haired, curvalicious beauty with big blue eyes and alabaster skin, Carrie is like one of those rivers whose depth stretches into infinity. You can actually see the wheels turning, thoughts churning, reflections forming in the quiet of her watchful eyes. She is extremely well-read, a veritable literature junkie, and a gourmet cook to boot.

Together with our merry band of misfits at the agency in Indianapolis, we had spent many an after-work happy hour lounging at the cozy dive bar down the street, popping champagne or downing good red wine. We usually ended up at someone's house, where any of the three fabulous cooks in our group whipped up a simple supper of brie, baguettes and seasoned, pan-seared scallops. It pays to have foodie friends. Those were yummy days.

Carrie and I forged our friendship during a key turning point in both of our lives. Our roads collided as she ramped up a new romance with the man who would eventually become her husband, and my relationship with my longtime boyfriend began to unravel.

We lived in the same city for only a year and a half—and our friendship didn't really blossom until maybe six months into that. Over 90 percent of our relationship has been via email. Since we're both writers, we can go months without actually speaking to each other, but through countless trials, we have been there for each other with supportive and heart-wrenching email missives detailing every thought in our heads. We dreamed of big things: publishing books, trekking the globe, producing our own TV shows and creating kick-ass marketing campaigns. We cried on each other's virtual shoulders during my broken engagement to my former boyfriend and her years of searching and self-doubt. We cheered each other on during my budding entrepreneurship and her brave leap into writing her novel. And as fate would have it, when I actually picked up a phone and called her to share news of my wonderful engagement to Paul, she informed me that Scott had proposed that same week. Sometimes, I wish we'd kept all of those emails. Reading them would be like tracking a civilization's evolution.

When Paul and I got married in April 2006, Carrie and Scott flew out to San Francisco to witness our wonderful wedding by the Bay. Two weeks later, we tacked a few days onto our Belizean honeymoon to watch them tie the knot at an intimate Key West seaside dinner party. Symmetry.

When Scott and Carrie are around, we all eat well. They can cook up a gorgeous *osso bucco* without breaking a sweat, and they annually travel to France to pursue gastronomic pleasures.

So during their visit to Seattle in early August of 2008, I made reservations for that Friday night at one of my favorite Italian restaurants in Seattle's Capitol Hill neighborhood.

My good friend Ursula was also in town. Ursula is a fit and sassy Australian with whom Paul and I had both worked at our last company. Outspoken, fiercely loyal and delightfully silly, Ursula was my cosmo-swirling buddy on many a Friday night during my single days. Of course, we're both good girls at heart so we also attended the occasional Sunday mass together and shared quiet dinners at home. One Christmas, Ursula took me to Sydney to celebrate with her boisterous and close-knit family, and we had a blast for two weeks. We both come from ethnic families and I was surprised at how similar in tradition, loyalty, and devotion to food her Lebanese family is to my Italian one. Her mother adopted me into her brood and led me along with her own three girls to Christmas mass, where we filed silently into the pew like ducklings, decked out in our prettiest skirts.

That weekend, Ursula stayed at our house, while Scott and Carrie luxuriated at their favorite Seattle boutique hotel. Ironically, Ursula had sat with Carrie and Scott at our wedding two years prior, so they already knew each other.

Perfect, I thought. We'll all go to dinner together.

The events of that weekend slowly revealed themselves to me in the months following. It was a long time before I could remember anything we'd done past dinner that Friday night.

I do remember walking into the restaurant. I remember a medium-bodied bottle of red wine, laughter and some delicious pappardelle. The details, however, are still a bit hazy. Paul went home right after dinner because he was exhausted, but I stayed out with Scott, Carrie and Ursula.

Still somewhat unfamiliar with my new city, I wasn't really sure where we could go for an after-dinner drink together. We wandered up Pine Street and I spotted a bar called Wild Rose with music spilling out the door and onto the sidewalk. Paying the cover and stumbling in, we looked around to see women gathered together in groups of twos and threes. It took us a moment, but we laughed as we realized I had chosen a lesbian bar to entertain my heterosexual out-of-town-guests. Ah well. We stayed put, but after all of the dinner wine, one cocktail in the bar caused a wave of fatigue to wash over us—especially our visitors from the eastern time zone—so we piled into cabs to go home.

By piecing together the events of the next day, I recall that Ursula and I hit Pike Place Market. The sounds of boisterous fishmongers and bustling tourists assaulted us. We meandered around bright, fresh veggie stands and miles of the most beautiful fresh flower bouquets you've ever seen: bright reds, yellows, greens, pinks and blues bursting before your eyes, and each arrangement more perfect than the next. The aromas of sweet chocolates, freshly baked pastries and homemade cheese mingle with the salty air wafting from Puget Sound. I love showing visitors the Market. It's a feast for the senses.

We wandered out of the market into some nearby shops, and she screamed in delight when we found a rustic spice store. Ursula had just started an online blog devoted to spices and cooking, so we spent a considerable amount of time sampling and sniffing from the barrels. I did not remember this side trip at all until I drove past the store, months later, and got a flash of recollection. When you are able to fill in a black hole in your memory, you get the same high as when you find that crucial jigsaw puzzle piece that fits. I think I actually clapped with glee.

Ursula left on Sunday and I prepped for a new audition at a different theatre company. A little spooked that I'd have a repeat of the last one, I did everything I could to keep my nerves in check, including light stretching, deep breathing and positive self-talk.

I headed out early to the cramped studio space in Capitol Hill. Climbing the rickety steps, my body warmed and my face flushed as the blood once again started rushing to my head, where a slow pounding started. Carefully breathing in and out, I made my way to the restroom.

"Okay, this is not going to happen again," I ordered my reflection in the mirror, as beads of sweat formed on my forehead. A few more deep yoga breaths seemed to settle the pounding and then I performed my little water-on-the-wrists trick. Miraculously, I felt my body temperature dip down a bit, and the blood rush subsided.

Shortly after that, with a touch of a lingering headache, I performed my monologue perfectly.

"I did it, babe!" I exclaimed to Paul later on. "I figured out how to cope with the nerves and blood pressure this time!"

Yeah, right.

Apparently my attempts that day were not as successful as I'd hoped. That night, I once again had my throbbing head stuck in a toilet, vomiting.

Paul found me passed out on the bathroom floor, but when he roused me, I convinced him I was exhausted and had just fallen asleep.

The next day, August 4, I was due to work at a client's office but I woke with the now familiar neck pain and that same wicked migraine squeezing my head in a vise. I knew I was going nowhere. After calling my client to let her know I wouldn't make it in, I tried to sleep. It was the only way to handle the stabbing head and muscle pain.

Paul usually takes the Microsoft Connector bus to work. Microsoft conveniently started this internal bus system a month after we moved to Seattle. The company sends out little buses to various neighborhoods to help ease employee commutes. It's completely free for employees, and the other side benefit is that they get to use the speedier carpool lanes when returning home during rush hour. We lived a few blocks from a Connector stop.

That day, however, Paul changed his plans.

"Why don't I take the car into work, in case I have to come back and help take care of you?"

"Don't be silly. You won't have to do that. I'll just sleep most of the day."

But he didn't listen. Thank God. Might be the only time I'll ever be thankful for that.

This day is still a huge black hole for me. I remember the intense head pain and the nausea. I remember Paul coming home midday so he could work from home and take care of me. He brought me chicken soup for lunch to ensure I ate something. I have a brief memory flash of me in my PJs, standing at the kitchen counter, slurping down the soup and valiantly trying to keep something in my stomach so I'd have something to throw up.

Then things go completely blank. At least for me.

Paul, my friends and my family, however, later filled me in on the horrific details that took place over not just the next twenty-four hours, but the next thirty days.

I believe things are worse for those who can clearly remember trauma than they are for those of us experiencing it firsthand. Our own memories often protect us from ourselves, but it's a lot harder to strike those images from the minds of the loved ones around us.

THE DAY I ALMOST DIED

I FOUND OUT MUCH later what had happened.

After making the soup for me for lunch, Paul went to my office downstairs so he could work. We have a three-story contemporary townhome, so my office and the front door are at ground level. The second level is an open floor plan of kitchen, dining room and family room, and then the bedrooms are on the top floor. I lay on the couch on our main level, trying to watch TV and silence the drill boring into my skull. At some point, I ran to the bathroom to throw up again. Since it's at the top of the stairs leading to the office, Paul could hear me retching.

He heard a loud thud and then silence. The dog started barking, whining and running in circles. Paul came upstairs to investigate.

I lay on the bathroom floor.

Collapsed and unconscious.

I imagine him springing into action like a superhero. He must have tried to revive me and when that didn't work, he had the presence of mind to call 911. God love him, he also called our good friend Barb to come help him.

"Maria passed out. The ambulance is on its way. Can you please come get Eddie?"

Barb did not even waste time asking questions. Still in her workout clothes, she ran from her house two blocks away to assist.

I love my friends.

Barb arrived to a frantic Paul, pacing and wide-eyed with fear. A fire department ladder truck happened to be nearby and arrived first on the scene, ahead of the ambulance. Seeing me laid out on the floor, ghostly pale as the paramedics worked on me, she started shaking.

"Has she overdosed?" the straight-laced EMT asked, shining lights into my eyes and poking and prodding various body parts.

"No...no, not at all," Paul stammered. "She's never taken drugs in her life!"

"Sir, maybe you were not aware...?" They tried to be tactful but I was showing all the signs of a drug overdose. The paramedics rifled through the Excedrin and vitamin bottles on our counter to be sure.

Our townhouse is impossible to find because we are up a steep stairway, behind a house and have no visible address from our street, so the ambulance was having a hard time finding us. Barb ran out to the back alley to wave them in but no one came. She ran back inside and realized Paul had ushered them in from the street below.

The paramedics couldn't get the gurney up our narrow stairwell, so they wrapped me in a sling and carried me down.

For all anyone knew at that moment, I was in a coma. Severe unconsciousness can point to brain damage or a possible stroke. With my brain basically "offline," the paramedics had no idea if major organs, such as my lungs, might start failing. Or, even worse, if my protective reflexes—like coughing or swallowing—were affected. Consequently, they focused on ensuring my system didn't physically shut down and that I could still breathe.

After they got me downstairs, they intubated me by threading a long plastic tube down my throat, and then bagging me with a valve mask on the way down to the ambulance. Hard-core sedatives must have followed after that, because I've learned that if a person regains consciousness with a tube down his throat, the first survival response is to rip it out—and that would be very, very bad.

I don't think anyone needs to see the one they love having a breathing tube rammed down their throat at top speed. Just picture all those old *ER* episodes and you'll know exactly what I mean. Freaking out, Paul tried to process where they were taking me so he could follow. Barb took Eddie, locked up and went home.

With its sirens blazing, the ambulance raced five miles to Harborview Medical Center, the only Level I adult and pediatric trauma center in the Pacific Northwest's four-state region. Everyone knows from watching the news that it's where gunshot and car crash victims from miles around are always sent.

On the way, the paramedics assessed me using the Glasgow Coma Scale[1]. This neurological scale assesses a head injury patient's consciousness level but is now commonly used by first responders for any acute medical or trauma patients like me. Specifically, it measures eye, verbal and motor responses. On its fifteen-point scale, anything below an eight suggests severe injury. In some cases, anything below a four is considered near death.

I was a three.

PART TWO

Life . . . Interrupted

Sleep, riches, and health to be truly enjoyed must be interrupted.

\- Johann Paul Friedrich

RICHTER, FLOWER, FRUIT AND THORN

The gem cannot be polished without friction nor man without trials.

\- Confucius

CHAOS, COMMUNICATION AND THE RALLYING OF THE TRIBE

I CAN ONLY IMAGINE what my husband encountered when he burst into the chaos of the emergency room. I was shocked to learn later that they let him drive himself there.

When I arrived at Harborview, the doctors whisked me into a CT scan to find out what the heck was going on. They immediately spotted a ruptured aneurysm on my right anterior communicating artery, which is located in my brain's frontal lobe. An *aneurysm* is a small bulge or "balloon" that stretches out from a weak spot in a blood vessel. Mine had burst, causing a specific type of stroke called a *subarachnoid hemorrhage* (SAH).

How is this a stroke, you may ask? A *stroke*, by definition, disrupts the brain's blood flow and damages brain tissue. Most people think of what's called an *ischemic* stroke, which is ninety percent of all strokes. In that situation, the artery is blocked or narrowed to the point that it severely limits blood flow. But a less common stroke is a *hemorrhagic* stroke like mine, where the blood vessel actually leaks or bursts.[2]

Because my aneurysm balloon had ruptured, it forced the blood to reroute itself—much like a reckless downhill skier into a normally off-limits area—into what's called the *subarachnoid space*.[3] With a name like that, you're likely to think of extraterrestrial spiders terrorizing the nether regions of the galaxy, but the subarachnoid space is actually located between the brain and the thin tissues that cover the brain.

What's a Subarachnoid Hemorrhage (SAH)?

No, I did not have spiders in my brain, despite the SAH's arachnid-like name, but it's certainly possible I may have imagined I did at some point.

However, a SAH is one type of hemorrhagic stroke. It may occur spontaneously—usually from a ruptured cerebral aneurysm, as mine did—or as a result of a head injury. My symptoms during the previous months had been a textbook SAH case; possible warning signs include a severe headache with a rapid onset (the "thunderclap headache" I experienced at the theatre audition), vomiting, confusion or a lowered level of consciousness, and sometimes seizures. The SAH "comprises 1–7% of all strokes and can lead to death or severe disability—even when recognized and treated at an early stage. Up to half of all cases of SAH are fatal and 10–15% of victims die before ever reaching a hospital. Those who do survive often have neurological or cognitive impairment." [4]

But at this point, I was still unconscious, so they had no idea what damage had been done. The CT scan merely provided physical confirmation that there was severe bleeding.

The scan showed a glowing white area in the front right center of my brain, where the aneurysm's bleeding originated. The blood extended outward into bright white trails and eventually surrounded the entire circumference of my brain where the subarachnoid space is located. The neurosurgeons—or "brain ninjas," as Paul came to affectionately call them—immediately stabilized me with powerful sedatives to both keep me unconscious and drastically lower my blood pressure to curb the blood from pumping so aggressively. Once it was under control, they scheduled me for the earliest possible surgery to repair the damaged artery.

There are two ways to stem an aneurysm, which was the goal of the surgery. One method is by cutting through the skull and clipping the aneurysm's neck shut, much like a clothespin. Or, in a slightly less-invasive manner, through *endovascular coiling*. Coiling involves threading several metal wires, one at a time, up through a catheter inserted into the femoral artery at my groin, through my blood vessels, and up into my brain. They get to your head through your leg…crazy, right? As doctors insert the wires into the aneurysm itself, they weave them together like a basket to disrupt the flow of blood into the aneurysm and to clot the bleeding. It sounds like a macabre sort of knitting, in my opinion.

I was a candidate for the coiling method simply because the aneurysm was the right shape (the neck was narrow enough to hold the coil firmly in place) and in an accessible location. In addition, my brain was pretty swollen at this point and the coiling procedure is less risky than opening up the skull when the brain is in that condition.

As Carrie later said, "The coil was platinum, naturally. Nothing but the best for you, babe."

What's A Coil?
I guess a platinum wedding ring just wasn't enough for me. Apparently, I needed this primo metal inside my brain as well. Doctors inserted a catheter (a small plastic tube) into my leg's femoral artery and navigated it through my blood vessels (the vascular system), up into my brain and then into the aneurysm itself. Tiny platinum coils are then threaded through that catheter and deployed into the aneurysm to block blood flow and prevent further rupture. The coils are made of platinum, a softer metal, so that they are visible via X-ray and remain flexible enough to conform to the aneurysm's shape.[5]

Paul must have been shell-shocked as he waited amidst the commotion of the busy ER for news. The doctors called him in to see me after they had assessed the situation. Dazed and staring at his unconscious wife hooked up to a ventilator, he tried to make sense of what the doctor said about my CT scans.

And as they prepped me for the surgery, I can only imagine Paul's horror when the doctor laid a hand on his shoulder and said, "We will try to save her life, Mr. Ross, but that's all we can do. We have no idea what she'll be like coming out of this." I cry when I think of him standing there, alone, as I was wheeled away. I'm his wife; I should have been there for him during that difficult time, but I obviously couldn't be. Memory was kind to me but not to him.

Crying in a corridor, Paul called my brother Michael in Columbus, Ohio, to tell him the news. Devastated, Michael agreed to serve as my family's central contact and spread the word to everyone else. He informed my other two older brothers, Patrick and John, and then got the not-so-fun task of notifying my close-to-eighty-year-old parents that I was in grave danger. Shocked and not quite sure what to expect, they all made immediate arrangements to fly to Seattle.

As the youngest of four and the only girl in my Italian family, I had my own private Jedi Council in my brothers. In a quirky twist, they are all six years older than me. Patrick was born in January and twins John and Michael in December of that same year. Quite a feat for our mom, who had tried to have children for eleven years before she literally hit the mother lode. I came along six years later to disrupt their GI Joe- and testosterone-fueled kingdom. My first act as new little sister was to cause the family dog to be given away when he started exhibiting aggressive behavior toward me as a perceived new rival. I'm sure if my brothers had been given a vote, they may have chosen the dog over me.

But later they became my protectors and my friends. Between the three of them, they taught me how to tie my shoes, how to do complex multiplication, and how to throw a punch correctly (not "like a girl"). As we grew, my parents often consulted my brothers about how to deal with me. Should they let me go out on that date? Should I be given a curfew on prom night? Since they were older than many of my friends' parents, our parents leveraged my brothers as a sanity check on what was really going on with kids my age, and I leveraged my brothers right back as a buffer when I thought my parents were being unreasonable. It was a great little set-up.

After my family learned of my precarious health situation, and my three brothers were descending into town like Caped Crusaders after seeing the Bat Signal, Paul enlisted our friend Guy to inform the San Francisco crew. He sent a mass email, and when another of our friends received it, he promptly dialed Ursula, who he knew was already in Seattle. She had inadvertently been left off the list in the chaos. Ursula called Paul to find out what had happened and told him she'd remain in Seattle for a few days to help before returning to San Francisco as planned.

Paul's next call was to his parents in Scotland. His mother immediately made plans to get on the next flight out of the country to be by his side. Then my lovely husband called one of my best friends, Becky, who was about five months pregnant and living in New York with her husband and toddler son.

Becky has been my friend since we met at orientation for our first post-college job as management consultants in Chicago. As I sat across from her in a room of strangers, I made a poor attempt to pantomime that she, Mary (another friend who would come to my aid) and I were all in the same division together. Becky thought maybe I'd gone off my meds as I made strange, circular gestures in the air. The three of us became fast friends and even roommates for a while. Becky is the reason I moved to San Francisco. After living a country apart—she on the West Coast and I on the East Coast and then back to the Midwest—she recruited me to come out and work for her San Francisco start-up in 1999, just in time to enjoy the tail end of the dot-com heyday.

Becky is truly the sister I never had. We are both the youngest in our families, both the only girls with older brothers whom we admire. She has her own gravitational pull. People flock to her energy and welcoming spirit, and she makes every single one of her friends feel like they are the most important person in her life. From what I've learned of her college days, she was president of every organization under the sun, and she kept this trend going into her professional life. Uber-connected and extremely extroverted, Becky has made introductions and connections for others that have resulted in lasting friendships, fruitful business partnerships, and even press coverage. With her bubbly attitude, dimpled grin and green eyes constantly crinkled with happiness, you just can't resist her charm.

Becky supported me through a multi-year, long-distance romance, a difficult but necessary broken engagement and various bad dating exploits during my twenties and early thirties. She's given me tough love, supportive love and motherly love, and she was delighted when I finally chose a normal, nice guy in Paul. Which is why she was shocked to hear from him directly that day.

"You need to sit down," he told her.

Her antennae went up. "I'm not sitting down, Paul. Tell me what's wrong. What happened?"

"Maria had an aneurysm. We're at the ER and she's going into surgery."

"I can be there this week. When do you need me there? What do you need?" Ever the organizer, she's planned birthday parties, baby showers and camping trips when the rest of us were too flighty to get our acts together.

Paul asked her if she could help him manage all the family and friends that were going to be flying in over the next several days. At the time, Becky thought I had merely discovered an aneurysm and that they were proactively operating on it before it burst. She had no idea that it had actually ruptured, causing the hemorrhage and brain damage. Adding further poignancy to the situation and a huge testament to her amazing friendship, an aneurysm had taken her own mother's life in 2003. When I had received that tearful, early-morning phone call years ago, I hopped the next flight to be by her side. Now, years later, here she was, flying out to another loved one taken down by an aneurysm but hoping this outcome would be better.

Becky notified all of our other mutual friends who were flung across the country. True to form as the master connector she is, she'd even kept the contact information of two close childhood friends of mine whom she'd only met once or twice. Becky coordinated travel plans for those who were on their way to Seattle from various states, including California, Wisconsin and Virginia. She blessedly took the burden off Paul at a time when he couldn't even think straight and barely remembered to feed our dog, Eddie.

After making these calls, Paul sat alone in the cafeteria for a few hours to wait out my surgery. Numb with shock and fear, I can picture him staring into space with a furrowed brow, pounding head and eyes red from crying. He didn't know what to think.

After a while, Guy and Barb made it to the hospital and sat with him in the deserted cafeteria to wait for news. They talked about me and, after hours of stress and tension, reassured themselves that I would be fine by finding some black humor in the whole situation. Paul was exhausted with worry by this point, so Guy made a call to Scott and Carrie that prompted them to extend their trip and stay on in Seattle.

After our dinner excursion on that previous Friday night, Scott and I had planned to meet after his video shoot at Microsoft that fateful Monday, since we were both slated to be on the company's Redmond campus, which is across Lake Washington from Seattle proper.

"I'll just plan to give you a ride back to Seattle with me," I had offered on Friday. He agreed.

That Monday morning, Scott went to the on-campus studio in Redmond, signed in at the front desk, and completed a day's worth of shooting. As things wound down, he called my cell phone and got voice mail. The session wrapped and he tried calling again. The same chipper, only-semi-business-like voice of Maria, asking callers to leave a message. Then he shot me a text: "Where r u?"

Scott went to the front desk and looked at the sign-in sheet. No Ross. No Marias at all, in fact. He asked the receptionist, who had been there all day, if an "unmistakable and very energetic redhead had passed by."

Nope, she said.

Something was amiss.

Scott's natural inclination and imagination might normally have taken him someplace morbid: to imagined car wrecks, bridge collapses, plane crashes, or alien invasions. But this time, he just assumed that my schedule had changed and that, sometime after 5:00 p.m., he'd get my call with a completely understandable and enthusiastic, "Oh, my God! I'm SO sorry, but this *huge* opportunity came up and…"

So Scott adapted, called a cab, and texted Carrie that I was MIA.

As he entered his hotel lobby, there, finally, was my caller ID flashing on his phone.

"So, what up?" he said cheerfully.

"Hi, Scott. This is Maria's phone, but it's not Maria," replied a male voice that was obviously not mine but confusingly not Paul's either. "I'm Maria and Paul's friend Guy, and I have some…well, it looks like bad news."

By the time Scott got his first inkling of the situation, he was back in the hotel room, where Carrie was sitting on the bed. As he walked in with the phone glued to his ear, she felt a nervous energy in the air, and within seconds she was trying to decipher exactly what had gone wrong.

All she heard was his side of the conversation. "Yes. All right. Which hospital? I understand."

"What is it?" she asked, but she was already crying, because she knew that whatever it was, it was life changing.

They sat in stunned silence for a few minutes. Then they called to cancel their trip home to Indy.

Meanwhile, back at the hospital, Paul, Guy and Barb sat in the eerie silence of the cafeteria until about eight o'clock that night. Waiting, hoping, praying.

Suddenly, Paul's cell phone rang. It was the nurse, telling him I was out of surgery, the doctors would come and speak to him soon and they just needed to know where he was. Paul told her.

The doctors walked up to the table and sat down. In calm yet confident tones, the neurosurgeon and his resident doctor told the worried bunch that I was still alive and that the procedure had been successful. I was in the recovery room but would soon be moved to the Intensive Care Unit (more commonly known as ICU), and once that happened, the doctor said a nurse would come get them to see me.

Paul exhaled in relief but still couldn't wrap his mind around it all. How had he ended up waiting in a hospital cafeteria for news on his wife's life, when a mere twelve hours ago, our lives had been fine? He simply trusted that nurses would be by shortly to bring him to my room. After waiting another hour or so, he got impatient and went up to find me in ICU himself.

Upon entering my private room, Paul sucked in his breath. I lay unconscious and surrounded by various blinking and scary machines. A nurse was at my beck and call at all times, watching and waiting.

"I was petrified," he admitted later. "You looked incredibly fragile."

A neuro ICU specialist then told him that he needed to drill a hole in my skull and insert a draining tube to flush out the blood and alleviate the pressure.

"Oh, yeah. Right. Of course," Paul responded. *Wait....what? Drill a hole in my wife's head?*

Paul later told me, "That was the point when things shifted from being bizarre and scary to becoming a series of routine check points. They were going to drill a hole in your head and I was expected to just accept that. After that, things that would normally have been extreme or strange simply became a normal part of the process we had to go through to make you better."

Carrie and Scott finally arrived at my room in Harborview's ICU and joined Paul, Guy and Barb. Tubes and wires stuck out of my frail body. Scott said later the scene was one of hushed tag-team comforting: Carrie and Paul alternately calmed each other, Guy and Barb calmed Paul, then Carrie. Then they alternated. Carrie couldn't tear her eyes off of the ventilator and, even now, years later, says it's not an easy memory to linger over.

"It's not like it is on television, with the breath just calmly going in and out. It's more...brutal. Watching your chest rise and fall in time to the whooshing sound—there was no doubt that the machine was breathing, not you."

Everyone agrees that the shared feeling was one of disbelief and unreality. They kept thinking it was a mistake and that I'd open my eyes and spout off a snarky comment. Is it weird to feel guilty that I am responsible for forcing this image and distress onto people I love? I know it wasn't my fault and I didn't ask for an aneurysm, but still, it's hard to swallow that I caused all that pain.

I am amazed at how news like this spreads and how my husband had the presence of mind over the next few days to review my email and online address books for names that looked familiar in order to let those people know. He tracked down my contacts through files, from notes strewn all over my desk and from incoming emails, and he quickly informed them as to what happened. The day after my aneurysm burst, I had failed to appear on a planned conference call with a potential corporate client. Luckily, Paul sent her notification when she sent a follow-up email. I'm sure that in a million years, "I had a brain aneurysm" was not the excuse she thought she'd hear.

That's the amazing thing. We all think our lives and work are so busy and important and we couldn't possibly take a break from them. We just keep running, running, running on the treadmill for fear it will all go to hell if we jump off. We check our voicemail every five minutes, we freak out if we forget our phone when we're running to the grocery store, and—God Forbid—we decide not to check email while on vacation. But when tragedy strikes, time just stops. And you know what? People adapt. Nothing, *nothing* is so important that it can't be worked around, no matter what anyone says.

...Unless, of course, they are performing emergency brain surgery.

MY TASTE OF INSANITY

Because I was still hooked up to the ventilator, I was heavily sedated in the early ICU days. As mentioned, they don't want patients waking up to find a huge tube crammed down their throat. It can be a little jarring.

After the successful coiling surgery and draining tube insertion, my next big hurdle was to breathe on my own. I was on Propofol, a highly potent sedative that can leave your system incredibly fast. You may remember it as the drug found in Michael Jackson's system upon his death. (Yes, he was supposedly using an ICU sedation drug as a "sleep aid.") Using a dial, the medical staff can control how fast you come out of sedation and slowly test the waters to see if you can handle breathing on your own. It's like a volume control for people. But don't get any ideas. I assume it's frowned upon to use it on unruly children.

Paul sat at my bedside and held my hand—and his breath—as they backed off from 10 cc's, then 5 cc's....and I immediately started coming to. He softly said my name, and I stirred, turning my head toward the sound of his voice.

This small ray of light was Paul's first sign that I might be okay.

The ventilator was then switched off and everyone watched. A monitor attached to my finger showed a red light that measured my red cell count and how much oxygen I was getting into my lungs.

My oxygen stats were a bit shaky at first. They were dropping too much and the doctors and nurses weren't sure if my lungs were able to take over. With bated breath, Paul clasped my hand tighter.

My oxygen level soon evened out and the medical staff confirmed I could breathe on my own. As a precaution, however, they decided to sedate me again and keep the ventilator in for one more day, just to let my brain settle down.

The next day, the whole dance was repeated. This time, Paul watched in feverish relief as they removed the tube completely. When you have no idea of the level of brain damage that has occurred, every basic bodily function is called into question. Thankfully, my lungs and my breathing all operated just fine.

So what the hell had happened to me?

The doctors believed that the initial headache in June had been a *sentinel bleed* in the aneurysm. This means the blood may have started leaking out of the blood vessel at that point. They couldn't tell us for sure after the fact, of course, but that was one of the working theories. Many people may never show any symptoms of an unruptured aneurysm if it is small enough.

The other theory was that the existing aneurysm had gotten so big, it was starting to exert pressure on the surrounding brain tissue, which triggered the headaches and pain. When the blood vessel wall weakened enough, it finally ruptured. That rupture caused blood to rush into areas of the brain where it wasn't supposed to be. It ruined tissue along the way, kind of like a knife slicing through butter.

This is one reason for brain damage. Another reason is that pressure builds up so much that it interrupts the brain's blood flow, which can lead to oxygen deprivation and tissue damage in certain areas. Since it was so soon after the rupture, the doctors had no idea what type of brain damage I had suffered—physical, mental or otherwise—or to what extent.

As part of standard ICU practice, I received many other sedatives. The month of August in 2008 is a complete blank for me, and I have just snatches of thirty-second memories here and there, as if I'm recalling a dream. Part of this was due to the intubation and sedation; part of it was due to the actual brain injury and short-term memory damage.

I later learned I said and did some pretty crazy stuff during that time and must have scared the daylights out of my family. Such symptoms can occur regardless of whether your brain injury is caused by an external force (referred to as *traumatic*), like a car accident, or from an internal source (referred to as *acquired*), like my cerebral hemorrhage. These are two different types of brain injuries, but they often share similar effects, depending on which part of the brain is impacted.

What's the Difference Between a Traumatic and an Acquired Brain Injury?

A traumatic brain injury (TBI) is when an external force—such as a gunshot wound, motor vehicle crash, assault, or when you fall and hit your head—injures the brain at any point after birth. My brain injury clearly wasn't due to a fall off the roof or speed racing, which meant mine was an acquired brain injury, or ABI. An acquired brain injury (ABI) includes all types of traumatic brain injuries, as well as brain injuries caused after birth by cerebral vascular accidents (commonly known as strokes), and loss of oxygen to the brain. Brain injuries that are present at birth or progressive in nature, such as Alzheimer's disease or Parkinson's, are not considered a traumatic or acquired brain injury.[6]

The amazing nurses educated my husband very well on what to expect in the first harrowing days in ICU as I became more alert. They warned him about possible brain damage and memory failure. They also told him I might show signs of what is informally called ICU psychosis: aggression, anxiety and even paranoia as a result of being in a sensory and sleep-deprived environment full of unfamiliar objects and people. ICU psychosis is a form of a technical term known as "delirium." I didn't know which way was up, what time it was, what day it was. My brain was frantically trying to piece things together and couldn't get them straight, which was compounded by my cocktail of medications and by the memory loss. Not surprisingly, patients with ICU psychosis often lash out at those closest to them when they feel trapped or afraid.

The brain is such a strange, wondrous place. With our intricate abilities as humans to dream, vision, imagine and pretend, I now understand why, when the wires get a bit fried, the whole system overheats and behaves oddly. Doctors say this ICU psychosis experience is very similar to what a person with paranoid schizophrenia goes through, neurochemically speaking. To be blunt and maybe a bit politically incorrect, I got to feel what it was like to be a crazy person for a little while.

As my roommate for many years, Becky knows this one strange fact about me: I hate movies in which something extraordinarily crazy happens to the protagonist and no one believes him, even when he tries to get help. We're talking about movies where a normal Joe Blow is mistaken for a spy and is kidnapped, interrogated and imprisoned, and no one believes he's telling the truth. Or movies like *The Net* with Sandra Bullock, in which her identity is erased by some bad dudes and replaced with a false one until they either get what they want from her or kill her first. She can't even go to the police for help because the records now show she is a wanted felon.

Watching these movies feels like drowning. I get a lump in my throat and panic rises in my chest. Why won't anyone believe them? What if I wander into a psychiatric ward and try to get out, and no one there believes I'm sane, and they just keep drugging me into submission?

Becky has long teased me about my frustration with such movies. Little did I know I'd actually learn what it really felt like. And, yes, it's as horrible as I'd always envisioned. People just won't *listen* to you!

One of my snatches of memory during this time was of utter panic. I thought I was late for a babysitting commitment, and I had no way of letting the parents know I was in the hospital. I must have pulled this notion from my high school experiences as the neighborhood babysitter. They say it's normal to experience this feeling of "missing something" when you have a brain injury—it's termed "agitation." It usually happens when you are coming out of the drug-induced haze and you're partially lucid. Your brain is trying to make sense of its surroundings, and it's a common ICU side effect as well. I've laughed over some bizarre stories with other brain injury patients who experienced the same thing. But I was absolutely convinced I was supposed to be somewhere. I pleaded with those around me to let me call and tell them where I was.

"But, Maria, who are you going to call?"

"Um....not sure..."

The thing about being brain injured but not actually certifiably crazy is that logic has a bizarre, unsettling effect on you.

Rationally, the explanation was that I was in such a state of confusion that I was taking input from a mix of dreams, reality, memories and even conversations I'd overheard in my sedated state. My brain was forced to create some level of understanding as it constructed its own reality in an attempt to get oriented to what was going on.

My family and friends were told not to confront me or tell me I was "wrong" when these incidents occurred. The nurses said all that would do is upset me more and put me into anxiety overload. Instead, my loved ones were told to simply calm me down by not necessarily playing along, but walking me through the logic of the situation.

For example, they might tell me, "Okay, Maria. We understand you're upset about missing this appointment. But who was it with?"

Of course, I couldn't answer. My brain would take a second to process that I had no idea who needed me and therefore maybe, just maybe, there was no commitment to be kept after all.

On another occasion, I believed I was late for a charity gala. When asked where it was or what I was planning to wear, the veil lifted just a little bit from my brain and I quickly realized there was no such event.

Whether I realized my mistake or not, my family was told to keep me calm and soothe me with, "Don't worry. We'll take care of that for you."

Elizabeth, a cherished bridesmaid and friend, flew in from Virginia to be with me. She is a cultured opera aficionado who appreciates high tea and perfectly wrapped presents—but who also gets in touch with her trashy side and can dish up juicy celebrity gossip every now and then. She and I enjoyed many a Saturday afternoon mani and pedi followed by a glass of wine when we were living in San Francisco. Shortly before Paul and I moved to Seattle, she relocated to Charlottesville, Virginia, home of her alma mater University of Virginia. Like us, she wanted out of the city and to finally buy a house. Her house, unlike ours, has a yard for her adorable little corgi, Cardi.

Given my penchant for fantastical ravings at this point, I almost gave her a heart attack on one of her hospital visits.

"Oh, my God, Elizabeth! Your dog sitter just called and Cardi ran away! What will we do?" She was totally sucked in for a little bit before realizing I wasn't thinking straight.

My friend Mary also fell victim to my pathological "lying." Mary and I had met in Chicago, post-college, and she now lives in Wisconsin, but she's a city gal through and through. Always sporting stylish clothes and expertly cut, thick black hair, I often envy her accessorizing skills. A petite five-foot-something (all I know is she's a tad shorter than my five-foot-four-inch frame), she's also a fit, former college cheerleader—which I was shocked to learn when I first met her, since she's somewhat reserved and so sleekly polished. Mary and I share a love for all things film and entertainment, and in our late twenties we even embarked on a slightly less dramatic version of a Thelma-and-Louise girls' driving tour around Ireland. She, Becky and I were the Three Musketeers at our consulting firm, represented by three petite yellow rubber ducks that Mary gave me the year I moved away. Those little reminders of our unbreakable tripod adorn my bathtub to this day.

When Mary and her husband, John, showed up at my bedside (again, I totally don't recall them being there at all), I fooled them with an eager, conspiratorial smile as I whispered, "There is so much going on around here, you have *no idea*!"

This was true, in a way. Poor Mary had no freaking idea what I was ranting about.

"The nurses and staff are involved in so much drama, it's like *Grey's Anatomy* over here!"

I've never even watched *Grey's Anatomy*. What the hell?

For a moment, Mary thought I'd discovered some juicy intrigue during the wee hours of the night. "You're normally fairly attuned to those types of things," she said.

Of course, this was all craziness. When pressed, I couldn't really explain this conspiracy theory about all the staff sleeping with and/or backstabbing each other, but she said later that I really enjoyed telling her about it and whispered everything in a very excited voice.

Could my mind simply have crossed wires between dreams, memories and imaginings? I think so. And nothing proved this point more than the *Gossip Girl* episode.

As my family and friends gathered around my bed in support and prayer, there were some lighter moments of utter boredom. Trashy magazines made their way into my room, and conversations turned to reality TV and celebrity gossip. What the hell else is there to do when someone is lying sedated in ICU, not quite out of the woods, but not in imminent danger either? There's a lot of downtime.

With all the discussions about pop culture and TV shows, it's not surprising that I came up with the craziest conspiracy theory of all, and one that now delights my friends and family when we recall it.

The evil plot? The hospital was a front for the TV show *Gossip Girl* (a nighttime soap opera I've never watched but which, I believe, is about rich teens in a Manhattan private school) and the nurses were all hired by the producers. According to my theory, the front desk staff was actually texting patient information to the show's writers and the stories would turn up on the air as plotlines. With this conspiracy theory firmly in place, I imagined a character resembling me would actually appear on the show with my name, my friends and my condition.

What was up with my mind's insistence that the staff were all in cahoots and often up to no good?

I've always been a pop-culture junkie and, as an actress, I love to dissect TV and film. But this was way beyond.

Apparently, I told this story to a few folks on several occasions and I'm not sure what their response was then. But I can recall the last time I told someone—Barb—about this evil plot and what it was like to really, truly, in my bones believe it to be true.

"I know this sounds crazy, Barb, but you have to believe me. The nurses are texting plotlines to the show's producers about us! Please believe me."

With her silence, I could feel her kind eyes looking at me with hesitation and a bit of sadness...which just made me shout all the more,

"I know it's completely crazy. I know it is. But it's true!"

After all those years of hating to watch movies in which the protagonist tries to get someone else to believe a fantastical and dire situation, I've learned I was right. It absolutely sucks when you desperately think something is true and you can't get anyone to believe your preposterous story.

I take it as a healing sign that at least I realized how zany the whole thing sounded. But to this day, I recall that moment of utter belief in what I was saying. It makes me see mental illness in a whole new light. It must be awful to hear voices or see visions and feel deep down in your bones that you actually saw what you saw and heard what you heard. And how helpless it feels to have doctors simply nod their heads in mock agreement but prescribe pills to make it all go away.

What did my family think when they heard these ravings and paranoid theories? It must have scared them to death to see me awake and talking with such ridiculousness coming out of my mouth. Did they wonder if this stage would pass? Or worry what it would be like if I was like this for the rest of my life?

At one point, Paul confided in Becky, "I can handle any physical challenges we might have to face. If she needs a wheelchair or a cane, or even if she won't be able to see again. We'll manage. But what if she's not herself ever again? What if her mind is gone? I don't know if I can handle that."

Becky—cheerleader, organizer, chick who gets things done—laid a hand on his shoulder and squeezed, "But you are handling it. And you will handle whatever comes. We'll *help you* handle whatever comes."

NOT-SO-PRETTY ROSES

AFTER DRIFTING IN and out of lucidity the first few days, I was being prepped for one of my many tests as Carrie stood by my side. I looked up at her.

"Where are the petals coming from? They're so pretty," I said dreamily, waving my hands in front of my eyes.

Carrie looked around perplexed. There were no flowers in my ICU room. "What are you seeing, sweetie?

"Rose petals. I can get them." I clutched at the empty air, trying to gather them up.

Scared, Carrie looked up at the nurse, who met her gaze and then ran to get the doctor. I sat back with a serene smile as I enjoyed the beauty I was seeing. Carrie said I was not frightened at all.

Ophthalmology hurried in to shine lights and poke at my eyes. At first, they gave a few false diagnoses: Some residents said it was reaction to the trauma and would heal in a few weeks; others said it could be due to shock. It was difficult to diagnose immediately because dilating my eyes to investigate it would get in the way of the neurological monitoring they needed to do.

In the end, they arrived at the right diagnosis. I had Terson's Syndrome.

Terson's Syndrome is a rare hemorrhage inside your eye that is caused by the subarachnoid hemorrhage (SAH) and the severely elevated brain pressure that I suffered. In SAH, only 13 percent of patients ever get Terson's Syndrome. It's usually only associated with the most severe SAH cases. To cause this type of damage, the brain pressure needs to get quite high, which means the risk of death is significantly increased.[7]

And yet, I was still here. I was still alive, despite these formidable odds. On the other hand, I was basically blind the entire time I was in the hospital. Blood had become trapped behind the lens but in front of the retina of each of my eyes and had impaired my vision. I like to say it's like pollution in the back of your eyeball. Or being stuck smack dab in the middle of a Monet painting. Or looking through a really, really dirty glass. You can make out shadows and broad shapes, and maybe some colors, but most of your vision is completely blocked.

Lack of vision probably added to my short-term memory loss and confusion about time, place and context. It's scary enough to lose your bearings. Heck, I thought it was 2003 and I was still living in San Francisco. But when you add that to not being able to process your surroundings or remember who you saw or what you were experiencing from one moment to the next, it can make you downright cranky. I bit people's heads off, snapped at Paul, and pouted like an adolescent child when my friend Ursula tried to stop me from getting out of bed to use the bathroom. I was draped in wires, with a draining tube sticking out of my head, and even a catheter in place for just such an occasion, but nooooooo....I was going to be independent, damn it!

Paranoia coupled with blindness in a foreign environment does not mix well. Your family and cherished friends are usually the ones to whom you feel safest unleashing the fury, and I was no exception.

But not everything was a *Gossip Girl* conspiracy or a fluttering of pretty rose petals. Sometimes my damaged brain filled in pictures for what it didn't see with intriguing but relatively innocuous images. For example, I could have sworn that the hospital was an old, three-story brick building. Mint-green marble tiles and black wrought iron banisters lined an old dark hallway reminiscent of an orphanage from the 1930s. All I was missing were Annie and the orphans. I held that image in my mind's eye for weeks.

In reality, the hospital was newly renovated and state-of-the-art, with comfortable and modern furnishings—even a nice balcony. Harborview is actually one of the best trauma centers in the country.

Did my mind envision a movie set from a forgotten film? Or an image I had created when reading a novel? I'm still not sure. But I remember being shocked during my first visit back to Harborview—with my full sight restored—for a post-discharge check-up. The building was all modern steel and glass, and clean, bright hallways. Nothing like what my imagination had created.

I've realized what a capable and detailed imagination I have. This idea of seeing what I wanted to see would come to both help and harm me as I worked to get back into my life.

THE FIRST HURDLE

I T'D BEEN A bumpy few days, but miraculously, I was still here. But the funny thing about brain injuries is that doctors can actually predict certain setbacks that will occur.

Carrie recorded much of those ICU days in a journal she kept by my bedside. Ever the writer, she bought a fuzzy orange journal with a playful blue monster on the cover. She used the journal to "talk to me" through her entries. While a few others joined in with an occasional note, it was mostly her way of processing this unchartered terrain.

Her first entry began:

August 7, 2008
It's so surreal. I want to email you or call you so I can tell you how you're doing. So instead, I'm doing what I do—writing to you when something's wrong.

Like clockwork, the first setback hit just four days into my ICU stay.

August 8, 2008
You're showing signs of a stroke. Your left eye wants to droop and they're concerned about a loss of strength in your left side. It's also affecting your speech a bit, which resulted in a little frustration. You finally en-un-ciat-ed and gestured in a very classically Maria way. Like so much of the last few days, it was both tough to watch and great to see. Tough to watch because we don't like to see you frustrated, but

*great to see because we're all living for the moments when the fog lifts
a little and we get a glimpse of you.*

Doctors initially disagreed on the cause of these stroke-like symptoms.
One doctor, Dr. Souter, quickly became my mother-in-law's favorite
because he was a Scotsman hailing from Inverness, the city near which my
in-laws live. How ironic to fly halfway across the world to be with your son
and daughter-in-law in a time of crisis, only to be met by someone from
your own backyard!

Dr. Souter correctly diagnosed my stroke-like symptoms as *cerebral
vasospasms*. A vasospasm is when your blood vessels constrict to protect
your body from blood it senses in the *cerebrospinal fluid* (CSF). CSF is not
just in your spinal column; it surrounds and "bathes" the brain to act as a
shock absorber and flush out waste. By squeezing shut, however, the vessels
can't get enough blood through to the brain—much like a traditional stroke.

Dr. Souter immediately ordered an angiogram to verify his diagnosis.
An *angiogram* is an extreme x-ray of your blood vessels. Medical staff
thread a catheter up your groin, through the femoral artery (like they do
for the coiling procedure), and inject a contrasting liquid that will show up
in the x-ray. The picture resembles a plate of spaghetti, and at Harborview,
they can even enhance it to appear in 3-D.

The point of an angiogram is to show the doctors if the blood vessels are
collapsed, narrowed or blocked. It's common after a cerebral hemorrhage for
your arteries to clamp shut as a defense mechanism some four or five days
after the initial incident.

Four days post-hemorrhage, sure enough, some of my blood vessels
constricted, causing a downgrade in my condition.

To solve the problem, they gave me drugs to open up the smaller vessels.
On the larger one, they performed an angioplasty. This procedure involves
attaching a small balloon on the end of a catheter to open the constricted
vessel back up again.[8] Kind of like pumping up a flat tire.

Post-procedure, my neural responses improved again and my fever
subsided.

So, crisis averted. For now.

THE NEW NORMAL

As WE ADAPTED to a new way of life while I lay in the hospital, Paul bore the brunt of it all. In the early days he was by my side constantly, his green eyes tinged with red and his face creased with worry from too little sleep and, most likely, even less patience. Crisis tends to rub our emotions so raw that the slightest touch can cause us to burst into flames or crumble like a cookie.

Becky revealed to me that she went straight to the hospital when she flew into town and made her way up to ICU. As she stepped off the elevator, she ran smack into Paul, who had just been told I was going in for my angiogram due to the stroke-like symptoms I was having. Setbacks like this are almost worse than the initial event, because just when you think you're out of the woods—*wham!*—you are hit with another obstacle. It's rather a cruel way to play with your emotions.

When the elevator doors opened and they unexpectedly greeted each other, Paul burst into tears.

For a brief moment, Becky thought I had actually died. But it was merely Paul's yo-yo emotions threatening to break him. My husband can be a little Scottish curmudgeon, with his sense of pessimism and dry wit. But most people soon realize that he has the kindest, most sensitive heart—and he's not a man who's afraid to show his emotions or vulnerability when pushed to the limit. When those tear-jerker ASPCA commercials come on TV and show mournful little puppy faces staring at you from behind bars, he lunges for the remote to change the channel just as quickly as I do.

Despite rare breakdowns like this, Paul remained as strong as a rock. I still hear tales of how he managed everything during this difficult time and I am in awe of him. He remained at my side through most of the ICU ordeal, and his bosses at Microsoft were extremely understanding and supportive. He did try to stay on top of emails as much as he could, so he "wouldn't get fired," he joked. He juggled so much during that time: all the visitors, his work, my ups and downs, our home, the dog, and his own emotional well-being. Paul was at the hospital every day for the 6:30 a.m. rounds to get reports on my progress.

As our visitors left town when I was out of the woods but still in the hospital, Paul got up at the crack of dawn, walked the dog, took him to all-day doggy day care, went to the hospital for rounds if he could, and then headed off for a few hours at work. Then, he'd come back and visit me in the afternoon when my therapies were done, then head back to pick up Eddie, maybe eat some dinner, sleep and start the whole thing all over again.

In the journal Carrie noted that this crazy schedule became our new "normal."

August 9, 2008
It's funny how things have settled into their own pace. These are the rules of the new reality—for now—and we're just figuring it out as each day presents itself. Paul describes it as a roller coaster: sometimes it's smiles and wanting ice cream, and sometimes it's pain and uncertainty.

The entire UW Medicine health system network, of which Harborview is a key player, is wonderful in that it subscribes to the philosophy of patient- and family-centered care. This means the experience and care is centered on the patient's needs. It seems obvious, but one way this translates into policy is that they let the patient decide who their "family" is (and isn't!). They also do not limit visiting hours.

Unfortunately for Paul, that meant I never wanted him to leave. He must have been thankful that the excessive fatigue common to brain injury meant that it wouldn't take long for me to tucker out and need my sleep.

This new reality also meant that our marriage roles were redefined. We'd always split chores like cleaning and whatnot, but Paul took on all of that, plus my role of dealing with the household finances. He had to handle our bills, which were all set up under my online banking login, not his. And he actually contacted my accountant to ensure my quarterly business taxes were paid on time for my consulting work, despite never having been involved with my business finances before.

It was more than just tasks, though, because the dynamics of our marriage also changed. Paul became my caregiver, not just my husband. I couldn't remember anything from one minute to the next—and I still couldn't even see. Even though the doctors would tell us both all the information about my condition and progress, Paul was the one who needed to remember it all. We were thankful that the hospital provided us with binders of information to take home, since we knew we weren't going to remember much of anything during those hazy and stressful few weeks.

This change in roles seemed obvious and right at the time. What else could we do? It wouldn't cause friction until later as we both got back into our "real" lives again.

THE SECOND HURDLE

SOMETIMES, WHEN YOU'VE been coasting along too easily and happily as I had been, life likes to throw you a curveball. And then follow it up with a few more for good measure.

I was still in ICU after surviving the initial aneurysm. The angioplasty had gotten me through the vasospasm episode with flying colors. My neural tests were improving, even if my memory was not. So, to add some spice, Fate decided to impishly sneak in and give me a bacterial infection.

We're talking the rubber gloves, isolation-type of infection. And not a very pleasant one.

Clostridium difficile is a lovely little infection commonly known as *C.diff*. It's found in hospitals and preys on the elderly and those with weakened immune systems, and it typically occurs after use of antibiotics. It can be passed by touch and is highly contagious, hence the rubber gloves and contamination room.[9]

C.diff causes severe diarrhea and can also lead to other intestinal conditions if not treated.

Good times.

This setback obviously delayed my transfer out of ICU. It was probably more of a pain to my friends and family than anything else, since I don't remember one single bit of it.

Becky had just flown in from New York a few days before—right as I was getting my angiogram. Nearly five months pregnant, she confirmed with her doctor back home that the *C.diff* would not harm her baby. With stringent hand washing and extra vigilance, she received the all-clear to stay in the room with me.

Of course, I kept forgetting the situation and why everyone around me was wearing masks and rubber gloves. It became just another one of those things in which everyone found a good laugh, another tiny moment where you seek the release of humor in a crazy situation.

Carrie wrote:

August 13, 2008
Funny thing you said to your brother John yesterday when you were told about the C-diff. He asked if you were sleepy and you said no. Then he asked if you were sad and you said yes. When he asked why, you said, "I'm bummed about my stool!" So cute!

Quieter days followed and the doctors said, "We like it when it's boring."

Paul continued to juggle work, our home, our visitors, our dog and me. Carrie noted:

Paul's a strong guy, but this is enough to break anyone.

Becky, who had also begun filling in entries, wrote:

His team at work is being very understanding. That's good, because I don't think he could leave your side for very long!

Thankfully, Paul had my family, our friends and his mom to lean on. They helped walk Eddie, prepare meals and shuttle people to and from the airport.

Even fairly new friends stepped in to bolster us up. Warren and Betsy Talbot, new friends we'd just made that summer—Paul and Warren worked together—arranged for a home chef to prepare meals and make sure everyone was well fed. Barb and Guy put my family up at their house. Other new friends Tim and Jill housed visiting friends.

The love and support around us was amazing and to this day still knocks the breath right out of me when I think of the countless acts—big and small—that people did...for us. It's both humbling and overwhelming. Not only does your own life stop when there is a crisis, but others willingly put their own lives on hold for you as well.

Carrie noted all of this emotional support in a touching journal entry:

August 9, 2008
I'm just keeping a very firm picture in my mind of the day that we talk—and, yes, laugh—about all of this. I may just tell you outrageous lies about what you said or did, so I can hear you say, "Oh, my God, I did not! Shut up." And I can tell you about the tremendous love that's around you. But, you know, I really believe you can feel it. Hang in there, Kitten."

She was right. I could feel it, even if I couldn't see it or remember it.

"WIGGLE THE TOES on your left foot. Very good."

"Push as hard as you can against my hand with your fist. Good."

"Raise your right arm, please. No, your *right* arm."

Brain injury or not, I've always been horrible telling my left from my right.

Carrie affectionately termed these constant exams "the ICU version of the Drunk Test." They typically roused me every hour so I could perform like a trained seal. Once, after being awakened for the umpteenth time, I turned to her and asked, "What the hell was that?! Sheesh!" and promptly went back to sleep.

Members of Team Maria drifted in and out of Seattle in the early weeks, and kind friends put them up all over town. My big Italian clan of parents and three brothers arrived a few days into the first week and camped out at Guy and Barb's house. Like champs, they navigated Seattle with rental cars and maps. It must have been nerve-wracking for them to fret, pace and support us—all while in an unfamiliar city thousands of miles from any familiar resources. My amazingly stoic and sassy mother-in-law flew in all the way from Scotland to handle Paul, handle Eddie (she's totally the pack leader with her own dogs; Eddie didn't know what hit him) and hold my hand. Early on, she mischievously tried to coax me into opening my eyes to come out of sedation.

"Come on, Maria. You have to see your nurse. He's just adorable." Poor Jess just stood there, his handsome cheeks blushing bright red. Carrie later confirmed that he was indeed "pretty yummy."

Tracy, another dear friend, flew in from Sacramento. A statuesque five-foot-ten, long-haired brunette with bright brown eyes and a dazzling smile, I'm sure she turned as many heads as my hot male nurse. Tracy and I partied lavishly in the San Francisco dot-com heyday and not only swirled way too much expensive Cabernet, but also went in on a Lake Tahoe ski house together a few years in a row. I joke that most of my prior credit card debt was a direct result of our friendship. What I love about Tracy is that she's got that Midwestern upbringing, and no matter our exploits, she's always an Iowa girl at heart. Gorgeous but grounded, sophisticated but sweet, she, like me, had done the singles scene for a while and had settled down with a wonderful, kind man in his hometown of Sacramento. I really missed being able to see her on a weekly basis.

As was to be expected, I asked people the same questions over and over. Becky said she felt like a rock star, because each time she came into my room, I greeted her like she'd just gotten into town. I sometimes guessed the month correctly when asked, sometimes not. And in the beginning, I needed reminding several times a day as to why I was in the hospital in the first place. One time, I said, "Oh wow. Bummer."

Something of an understatement.

Becky took a stab at writing a few journal entries to record my confusion:

August 14, 2008
You always get a bit confused when you're sleepy. You just asked Paul what time you are going home tonight. He had to tell you that you were staying for a few more nights. Earlier, they were asking you your questions again and you got everything right—name, year, president— except....the month. You REALLY want it to be February! However, we just discussed that it wasn't February, so you were trying to deduce which month it was. You guessed June.

The doctors just came by and said that your "spec" scan was improving! That's the one where they inject you with this radioactive dye and they scan everything to see what's going on (again, not the medical explanation). Anyway, that's really good news.

August 15, 2008
You had a bit of a rough night last night—fever, and the incision in your head was "leaking," so they had to do two rounds of new sutures

to fix that. But all in all, you are doing really well. Today was the first day the docs talked about "timelines"—when to remove the tube in your head, when to move you out of ICU, etc. All good signs, sweetie.

As assessments continued, the doctors watched to see if my body would take over some critical functions as they weaned me off various machines. When they prepared to remove the head drain, they clamped it first to see if my body could handle the job on its own. Paul wasn't sure if my increased confusion and sleepiness was a result of this change, or if that was just a sign that bits of my memory were coming back.

He wrote in the journal:

You were very confused a couple of times today, which I'm interpreting as bits of your memories coming back and you are trying to interpret them or sort them out. For example, none of my cousins have anything to do with horse racing!

No, not *his* cousins. But my mind must have caught a glimpse of the forgotten fact that my own cousin used to be a jockey and raced professionally. Maybe I was fighting my way back to the surface after all.

They had to make sure my head pressure was stable, so Paul sat monitoring it for hours at a time. Those readings, along with my CT scans, helped the doctors decide whether or not to remove the head tube completely. The drain was finally removed on August 18.

I have another snatch of memory from this time period, although this one's a doozy: Thirty seconds of an intense, searing pain cutting into the top of my head, while I screamed and cried and squeezed the life out of Paul's hand. They had removed the tube but, unfortunately, the numbing injection for the stitches did not take the first time. Given the choice to endure another painful shot that would prolong the pain, or to just grit my teeth and bear the short-term suturing agony, I chose the latter. I felt the needle going into my head and I can see this moment in my mind's eye as clear as day. I still can't believe I was strong enough to bear that pain, but it makes me proud in a twisted sort of way. That should have been my first clue that I was going to conquer whatever might come.

Carrie revels in researching on the Internet, poring over articles and learning as much as she can about unfamiliar situations. Thank God. A former editor, she observes and ponders every foible, every charm, and every drama like a gifted psychologist. This skill allowed her to slip seamlessly into her role as patient advocate: asking questions, taking notes, smacking down a nurse who almost gave me the wrong IV, admonishing a resident who was not supposed to move my precisely-angled bed, scanning websites and devouring books by Oliver Sacks. With this kind of firepower in my corner, things could not really go anywhere but up.

Graduation! On August 20, sixteen days after being admitted, I was moved from ICU to the neurosurgery ward. Gingerly, I took my first steps in over two weeks. Bracing myself against a walker, surrounded by cheering supporters, I placed one wobbly, atrophied leg in front of the other and managed a flight of stairs to the kitchen as they helped me make a cup of tea. Not exactly the marathon—and it would be a while before I could tackle my daily thirty-minute walks with Eddie—but it was surely a start. Everyone was so proud of me.

On that day, Tracy wrote:

You were out of bed and walking with a walker. When someone asked if you wanted to stop or keep going, you of course said, "Let's keep going." That's our Maria.

As the days passed, medical staff did daily neurological assessments, sometimes multiple times a day. They asked me a series of questions to see where I was from a cognitive standpoint. While I could have conversations when I was alert and awake, I still didn't always have a firm grasp on reality. But I think my friends and family enjoyed the barrage of questioning more than I did, especially Tracy:

They started a lot of testing and assessment for future therapy. Lots more questions followed, the first being 'Does a cork float?" I wasn't sure on this either. We just drink the wine. We don't bother putting the cork in water!

Over the course of my hospital stay, Paul, along with everyone else, turned to humor as a coping mechanism. He invented his own battery of memory tests. That fall, two prominent men made headlines: John Edwards and Brett Favre. John Edwards' scandal involved a secret affair. Brett Favre, the famous Green Bay Packers quarterback, went to play for the NY Jets. As I'm a big football fan, this bit of news mattered to me because I loved Brett Favre and I'm a Jets fan.

Each day, Paul asked me, "Do you remember what I told you about John Edwards? Do you remember what I told you about Brett Favre?" And each day, I forgot. You know that movie, *50 First Dates*, with Drew Barrymore and Adam Sandler, where each day he has to woo his girlfriend all over again because she suffers from having no short-term memory? Yeah, it was kind of like that.

"Shut up! No way!" I would exclaim in shock. Every single time.

"Never gets old," he joked. But Paul's amusement masked a nagging worry that I might be like this for the rest of my life.

In the vast blackness of a month entirely lost to my memory, I know there were glimpses of the old Maria that offered hope and comfort to everyone, just as much as there were some scary setbacks.

Even in my ramblings, I itched to be busy, telling people the location of things that I thought I needed from home (I didn't), or asking what I needed to be doing (nothing). My mind reeled off an ambitious to-do list on auto-pilot, even though none existed. Not all of it made sense, but everyone took it as a good sign that I wanted to be kicking ass and taking names again, especially Carrie:

August 9, 2008
We're trying to sort out a good pillow/position/bed height combo because of your neck pain so you're getting jostled quite a bit. During one of the jostles, your gown slipped a bit and you said, very distinctively, "Well, shit," and yanked it back up. Little victories, tiny friend...little victories.

THE THIRD HURDLE . . . LUMBAR PUNCTURES SUCK

Aᴺᴰ ᴛʜᴇ ʜɪᴛꜱ just keep on rolling. Who was it that said bad stuff happens in threes? This would be an important lesson I would learn throughout my recovery: sometimes a step forward means three steps back.

Tracy left on August 21 and Carrie flew back from Indianapolis to be there for me and Paul again. I imagine I was like a very well-loved baton or cherished stuffed animal, being passed off from one family member or friend to another. That just makes me feel so warm inside.

Carrie hadn't seen me since that first week in the hospital, when things were really dicey. She had a great perspective on how much progress I had made since then:

August 24, 2008
I got in Thursday to what was a whole new Maria. And by that I mean it was my old Maria: Funny, sharp, blowing Paul shit. It was literally astonishing to see you sitting up (no head drain!) and we went for a walk yesterday. I guess I missed you being outside today, but I did see (gasp!) pictures. Yes, someone finally took pictures of you. Sorry!

Part of treating cerebral hemorrhages like mine is to focus on preventing another rupture or rebleed. The ICU constantly monitored such vital signs as heart rate, blood pressure, respiration and temperature. The medical staff also noted my alertness, movements and speech[10], as well as the neural tests they gave me every hour or so. Such tests are designed to assess if I was alert and oriented to four things: place, time, person and situation. The staff asked my name, the date, where I was and what I thought I was doing at that precise moment. (Answering your test questions, duh!)

Later, other mental status tests were used to track cognition. Could I remember lists of short words, or track a conversation? The idea was to see if my mental alertness was changing over the course of days or weeks. With such constant evaluation, my medical team could then spring into action and course correct as needed, like the "medical ninjas" they are.

One physical metric over which they kept watch, especially in the early days, was my *intracranial pressure* (ICP). An increase in your ICP could indicate that too much cerebrospinal fluid (CSF) is building up and putting dangerous pressure on your brain and spine. Think of what happens when you overfill a water balloon and you'll get my drift.

Just like an airplane cabin does, your CSF regulates itself to the correct pressure to keep the inside of your body in balance.

At least, it should.

When my ICP spiked, this was bad news. They performed several spinal taps (also known as lumbar punctures) during my stay to both measure it and drain any excess CSF.

ICP? CSF? OMG!

Why on earth was the medical staff measuring so many acronyms for me in ICU? Increased intracranial pressure (ICP) is a rise in the pressure inside the skull that can result from or cause brain injury. An increase in intracranial pressure is a serious medical problem. The pressure itself can damage the brain or spinal cord by pressing on important brain structures and by restricting blood flow into the brain. Increased ICP can be measured either via spinal taps or directly, by using a device that is drilled through the skull or a tube (catheter) that is inserted inside the brain.[11]

Increased ICP could indicate a rise in cerebrospinal fluid (CSF) pressure. CSF surrounds the brain and spinal cord and cushions everything, kind of like a shock absorber. The fluid also brings nutrients to the brain and removes waste from the brain. Normally, CSF moves through areas of the brain called *ventricles,* then around the outside of the brain and the spinal cord. It is then reabsorbed into the bloodstream.

Brain traumas can cause an increase in CSF production and your body just can't absorb it all, thus causing the fluid to dangerously build up too high, as it eventually did with me. This condition is called *hydrocephalus.*

I'm glad I don't remember the spinal taps because they supposedly hurt like nothing else in this world. They jab a large needle into the base of your spine and draw out fluid. Not fun. Paul hated watching me cry in pain during these procedures. When he was preoccupied doing something else during what would be a particularly rough one, Ursula stayed by my side and gave the surgery team the nod to begin.

"Remember your bachelorette party at the Ritz Carlton Half Moon Bay?" she asked, distracting me from the pain. "Tell me what your favorite part was."

Gritting my teeth and squeezing all feeling out of her hand, I recounted how much I enjoyed all of us girls chatting around the beachside fire pit and our glorious spa massages. As I gulped for air and tears sprang to my eyes, Ursula prodded me to keep talking. She caught sight of Paul outside the curtain. Locking eyes with him, she nodded that everything was okay and I was getting through it.

The spinal taps helped alleviate the pressure temporarily, but the CSF still re-accumulated every time. Doctors determined my body could not effectively reabsorb this dangerous build-up (a condition known as hydrocephalus) so more drastic measures were needed. I was swept into another surgery to implant a shunt into my head. The shunt's valve was now regulating the fluid in my system on an as-needed basis, so no more lumbar punctures were required.

Of course, the shunt is now in my head forever and you can feel the ridge along the right side of my head. My brother John is afraid to touch it to this day, in case it's an on/off switch and I will suddenly "power down" if it's pushed too hard. The device lives in my skull and a tiny tube snakes down behind my right ear, crossing over the front of my neck and down the center of my chest, where it then drains any excess fluid into my abdomen.

After the successful shunt surgery, staples dotted my shaved scalp. I must have looked like Frankenstein. The head scar still lives underneath all of my now-grown hair and a small incision scar appears to the right of my belly button where they adjusted the catheter.

It doesn't set off airport alarms or anything like that. In fact, I hardly know it's there unless I sleep awkwardly and put too much pressure directly on it, or a masseuse freaks out about the tight muscle snaking its way down my neck. "That's a shunt tube," I have to warn her, or she may try to massage it out. I do, however, have to get the valve recalibrated with a magnet after an MRI.

What is a Shunt?

Doctors treated my hydrocephalus (excess CSF build-up in the brain) with a common treatment, which is called shunting. A shunt is a flexible tube that is surgically inserted in the operating room. A shunt redirects the flow of CSF from the brain to another part of the body where the fluid can be absorbed. The shunt is usually placed from the brain to the abdominal cavity. The tubing carrying the CSF runs under the skin from the head to the abdomen, just under the stomach.[12]

Performed in an operating room and with the patient under general anesthesia, the surgery takes about one and a half hours. Medical staff first shaves the patient's hair behind the ear. A doctor then makes a surgical cut in the shape of a horseshoe (U-shape) behind the ear, as well as another small surgical cut in the belly. After drilling a small hole in the skull, doctors pass a small thin tube called a catheter into a ventricle of the brain. They place another catheter under the skin behind the ear and move it down the neck and chest and, usually, into the abdominal cavity or chest area. The doctor may make a small cut in the neck to help position the catheter. A valve (a fluid pump) is placed outside the skull but beneath the skin, somewhere near the ear—in my case, above my right ear. The valve is attached to both catheters on either side. When extra pressure builds up around the brain, the valve opens, and excess fluid drains out of it into the belly or chest area where it can then leave the body. This helps decrease intracranial pressure. In newer shunts like mine, the valve can be programmed to drain more or less fluid from the brain.[13]

This unexpected operation set me back a few days from transferring to in-patient rehab, which had been targeted for August 25. I even had my bags packed and was ready to go into the next phase of my long road to recovery: grueling daily sessions of physical therapy, occupational therapy and speech therapy. The doctors felt that doing in-patient therapy for a few weeks would actually help me recover faster and heal more quickly once I got home.

This had been the plan before my ICP spiked so high, of course. But once we passed this hurdle, a bed opened up at University of Washington Medical Center (UWMC), a sister facility of Harborview located a few miles away. I was to be transferred there over Labor Day weekend.

The next stage of my recovery was about to begin. From this point forward, I have active memories of what was going on around me. I had lost a month of my life, but I was on the long road back.

HAIR TODAY, GONE TOMORROW

ALL MY LIFE, I have been referred to as "the little curly-red-haired girl."
Kinda like the gal Charlie Brown had a crush on, or so I'd like to think.
My hair has always been an extension of my identity. My signature. While I
sometimes hated what I perceived as my frizzy, "weird" hair as a kid, it was
also my ticket to standing out in a crowd.

As a child actress in NYC, I often nailed parts with my unique look.
Deep chestnut eyes and thick, long locks of flowing auburn curls were
not things I fully appreciated in my awkward teen years. I was too busy
believing I was the scrawny, little ugly duckling. But *Pretty Woman* came
out as I was entering college and Julia's big red hair looked a heck of a lot
like mine (it was 1990, after all, so B-I-G hair was all the rage). Suddenly,
guys were like, "You look like Julia Roberts!" Note: *I don't*. But it was a
nice line anyway.

Perfect strangers have come up to me in the street and asked me
where I got my hair permed. It's natural, I'd tell them, only to be met with
wistful envy or outright hatred. As a full-blooded Italian with both sets of
grandparents from Southern Italy, being a redhead made me even more
exotic (although there are quite a few redheads running around Italy).
When people asked how a pure Italian ended up with fair skin and red
hair, I'd quip, "Well, Italy *has* been invaded by everyone at some point or
another."

Of course, we all want what we can't have, right? I longed to have
straight, sleek hair. Hair that looked "together" and polished rather than
making me look like a disheveled cat lady. As an adult, I sometimes blow
dry my hair straight, just to shake things up. I had chopped off my long,

layered curls only twice in my life: once, in the sixth grade, when my mother's poor advice to a hair dresser resulted in me looking like a boy, and then in 1997, when I experimented with a just-past-chin-length look. Both cuts made my curls spring out even more stubbornly than before. I looked like a poodle. Longer hair was a much better look for me.

Why am I going on and on about my hair? Because it was a core part of my identity and something that made me...well, *me*.

When tasked with saving my life initially and inserting the draining tube into my head, the doctors had to do what they must do. They shaved some of my hair off on the right side of my head and then had to shave even more when they inserted the shunt. Blind, I was spared seeing this monstrosity. Every single one of my friends stated that the most shocking aspect of seeing me at the hospital was how small and frail I looked without my hair. Like I was a shrunken voodoo head lying in a sea of white sheets and tangled wires.

A close friend summed it up best: "I thought at the time that your hair was a symbol of your energy and vivaciousness and, like Samson, if they cut it off, you would lose some of your powers!"

So there I was, not aware of how ridiculous I looked with one half of my long hair tied into a messy braid and the other half completely shaved off. Some people said, "I can't believe they did that to you!" But I'm actually more grateful that the doctors were in the business of saving my life, not styling my coif.

One of my memory flashes is of a conversation with Paul and my friend Mary, right before moving to in-patient rehab. Paul and I debated what I should do with my hair and if I should cut it all off or not. Mary noted later that it was pretty clear that I had no idea what I looked like or how much of it was gone.

"Mary, can't you just part it on the other side or just style it somehow to cover it up?" I pleaded.

No way was my stylish little Mary going to give her friend a ridiculous-looking comb-over.

There was nothing to be done but cut it all off and let it grow back evenly.

After some convincing, I finally relented and Paul fetched a pair of scissors from a nearby nurses' station. I actually remember this tiny little vignette, perhaps because it was so traumatic. I could feel Mary holding my pigtail while Paul hacked away, hearing the "crunch, crunch" as the scissors worked their way through my thick hair. Thank God I was blind at the time.

It was a mess, Mary told me later. I had tufts sticking out all over. She took pity on me and tried a few touch-up snips to even it up. An improvement, but still not very good.

A few days later, our friends Warren and Betsy Talbot came to visit me in the rehab ward. Warren, a bespectacled lover of a good beer, photography and dinners with friends, was a co-worker of Paul's. Turned out his spunky wife Betsy, with her infectious laugh and signature orange scarves, and I traveled in the same tight-knit Seattle entrepreneurial community and knew a lot of the same people. We had just started becoming "double date" friends when this whole madness began. I asked them if they would take my ponytail, which I still had in hand, and donate it to Locks of Love, a charity that makes wigs for cancer survivors. They kindly agreed and, not having anything else in which to carry it, settled on a plastic Hazardous Materials bag they rummaged up at the nurses' station. Betsy said it was so strange carrying my hair in a haz-mat bag, and it just reinforced her image of my lost powers even more!

Weeks later, after eye surgery, I was able to see enough out of one eye to look at myself in the mirror for the first time. It was so shocking, I actually forgot to breathe. By that time, my hair looked like Natalie Portman's shaved do from V for Vendetta, and I, like everyone else, was amazed at how small my head now looked.

Tears welled up as I stared in the mirror that day for the first time: my left eye was still red and swollen from eye surgery, my face was pale and gaunt from all the weight loss and my hair—my signature, my trademark, my one pride and joy—was hacked to bits. I realized for the first time what a tiny little "pea head" I had hiding under all of that hair. I felt so small, like part of me had disappeared.

Who was I if I wasn't the feisty curly-red-haired girl anymore?

I guess I was going to have to find out.

Whoa, I thought. I have a helluva long way to go.

THE ROAD TO REHAB BEGINS

MY MEMORIES FINALLY began to take shape again Labor Day weekend, when I was transferred from Harborview to University of Washington Medical Center (UWMC), a sister hospital in the same UW Medicine health system network, for in-patient rehabilitation. How lucky am I that these hospitals, less than six months later in 2009, were nationally ranked for their rehabilitation care?[14] Again, fate stepped in and landed this blessed resource less than five miles from my house.

My brother Michael had come back to Seattle a second time, in part because he'd already had tickets to visit us for Labor Day. On transfer day, the Harborview staff apparently "lost me" for a while. Some miscommunication caused me to be moved to a ward upstairs, and when the ambulance drivers came to get me from my old bed, I was gone.

I vaguely remember not knowing where I was and envisioning being at the very end of a long row of curtained hospital beds, like an intake area of some sort. Tentatively, I called out but no one heard me—or so my memory tells me, but who can really trust that? I couldn't see, I had no idea where I was or where they had put me, and my heart started pounding in panic.

I called out one last time, "Michael? MIKE?!"

Finally, I heard him answer from what sounded like the end of a long corridor. "Mi? MIA?!" Michael has used this affectionate nickname since I was a kid.

Relieved, I let out the breath I'd been holding as he arrived at my bedside. "You found me!" I exclaimed.

He laughed. Later, he told me he spotted my shaved little pea head, lost in a sea of pillows and blankets as I frantically called out to him and scanned the room but saw nothing. "You looked so small in that bed, I wanted to cry," he said.

Spending two weeks in in-patient rehab at UWMC was a bit like being at the Canyon Ranch Spa. I had constant activities with my therapists, all meals were provided and I got to sleep in. No massage or poolside lounging, though. Ah well. With my vision problems, a girl could dream, couldn't she?

Now that I was more aware of my surroundings and my memory was starting to solidify from one day to the next, I really started feeling the fatigue that accompanies many subarachnoid hemorrhages. Up to three-quarters of SAH survivors report excessive fatigue, feeling drained, or experiencing daytime sleepiness for months—even years—to come. For about one-third of them, it may be permanent.[15]

And it's not like we're talking about training for a triathlon either. Normal, everyday activities like walking, talking and getting in and out of the shower can just drain you. Combine this with my brain working overtime to overcome the new cognitive deficits and I was often completely wiped out, both mentally and physically. For some patients, this type of fatigue can likely be caused by such medical conditions as anemia, abnormal blood sugar levels, or poor nutrition. But it can also be caused by insomnia, depression, lack of activity, or just your general emotional state. Being in the hospital really is not the best place to be when you're trying to get well. I couldn't go a whole day without a nap or two.

The goal of in-patient therapy was to get me mobile and help build my stamina and endurance. It was also a way to assess how much in-home care I'd need after discharge.

The schedule was relentless. Every weekday, I had three types of therapy. The first was occupational therapy (OT), which helped me conquer activities of daily living, or ADLs, as the lingo goes. This includes the basics, like grooming, bathing, dressing, making coffee, doing laundry, and general mobility. OT assesses whether I'm safely able to physically and cognitively handle these tasks independently. My occupational therapist also helped create cues and aids to make these jobs easier. OT is all about helping you do everyday tasks and function in your world.

OT is the therapy that made me feel the most helpless. I mean, really, they have to assess if I can take a shower by myself? I'm a business owner, for chrissakes! But what really made the tears spring forth was the fact that I did need someone to help me or at least be present so I didn't fall. I kept telling myself this was only due to my sight issues and would not be a problem much longer...but what if I was wrong?

The second daily therapy session was physical therapy (PT). This focuses on a person's strength, stamina, and balance. I liked PT because it made me feel like I was working out again. Katie, a good-natured, athletic-type with short brown hair and glasses, was my awesome physical therapist. Under her straightforward and patient guidance, we went to the gym and worked out. Where once I used to kick ass in a one hour spinning class, I was now proud of myself for doing three overhead lifts—with a two-pound weight. O, how the mighty have fallen.

But I craved the exhaustion from this physical activity because I knew I was making progress. Katie and I tested how many flights of stairs I could handle: three was our goal. She tied a little harness around my waist to protect me from falling, since my weakness and bad vision made for a double whammy. I have a photo of Katie leading me down a long flight of stairs, like a horse on a tether.

Our workouts took us all over the hospital, which was like an enchanted adventure since I couldn't see. I had no idea where the outdoor Healing Garden was in relation to my room but it felt like we trekked miles to get there. She could have run away and left me there and I'd have no idea how to find my way back. We often had to switch elevator banks to get to different parts of the hospital and I felt like Hansel and Gretel trying to see if I could remember the way back again without breadcrumbs. But my damaged short-term memory made this an impossible task.

Speech therapy (ST) was up next. You might think this applies only to stroke victims who can't speak, but ST covers treatment for memory difficulties, problem solving, concentration and even general use of language.[16] This therapy was the most frustrating, because I knew I might need some help but I wasn't sure what the outcomes were supposed to be. She read me short stories and then asked me to recount the story and some of the details. This seemed too easy to me and I felt insulted and belittled. Paul told me later that I was actually not very accurate at first but I got better as time went on. But, at the time, I felt like I was being misjudged. The type A performer in me did not like getting low marks from anyone.

"She thinks I'm stupid!" I cried into the blurry air, shouting somewhere in the direction of Paul. "When she asks me stupid questions, it means she thinks I'm an idiot. What do they think is happening to me if they are asking me things like, 'What is the name of the main character of the story?' I mean, really!"

Paul sighed. He was getting used to these emotional outbursts. These days, reason and logic didn't make me—the emotional raw nerve that I was—very happy. "She's just testing to see if you know the information. If you do, that's great. That's what we want!"

"She's patronizing me! No one here respects me. I'm still smart, right? I know I am!" I lashed out, more to convince myself than anyone else, and soon collapsed into tears. I couldn't see how these seemingly insulting questions were helping in any way. I left the speech therapy sessions feeling frustrated and no closer to achieving any goals.

Poor woman. I didn't realize how many different areas she could help me with.

Looking back, I think part of it was due to denial—and somewhat to ignorance—about what my longer-term cognitive issues might be. I thought I was fine, because I couldn't yet see what challenges awaited me once I got back to my real life.

AFTER THE EARLY September move to UW Medical Center (UWMC), I scored an appointment with retinal surgeon Dr. James Kinyoun. An older gentleman with a hearty laugh and an easy but direct manner, I immediately felt like I was in the right hands and would get some answers. He described Terson's Syndrome to me in detail—taking hold of my hands and having me feel a plastic teaching model of an eye as he did so—and told me it was temporary: my retinas would clear out on their own as my body absorbed the blood. But that could take ten months to a year.

How would I be able to complete rehab, get my strength back, walk, take care of myself, and get back to work?

Luckily, I was deemed a good candidate for a *vitrectomy*, which is the complex surgical removal of the vitreous gel from the middle of the eyeball. Put another way, they go in and clear away the debris so you can see. They replace the gel they remove with either a silicone oil or gas to restore your eye's normal pressure. Obviously, this needs to be performed by a skilled retinal surgeon and I was lucky that Dr. Kinyoun is one of the best. Once again, Paul and I told each other, "If you have to have a brain aneurysm, I'm glad it's here."

But surgery would not happen until after my hospital discharge. And he was only going to do it on one eye—my left eye—so I could at least function and make progress with my rehab therapies. Ideally, doctors prefer the eye clear up on its own, which is what they would let the right eye do.

For the next few weeks, until surgery, I remained blind.

The nurses kindly taped tactile prompts to my call button and TV remote. Paul filled out my food choices each day for the next day's meals since I couldn't read the menu. My physical therapist showed me how to make my way down the hall by grazing the wall and learning to feel and count the open doorways to find my room. She also showed me how to grope for the big silver button on the wall that automatically opened the ward's swinging doors. Because I could make out big shapes and obstacles, I achieved some mobility, but I wouldn't say I was sprinting through the hospital.

Trapped in the hospital with not much else to do, I couldn't read a book or a trashy magazine or even do a crossword puzzle. Paul loaded up some audio books for me on my iPod, but then I always had the issue of seeing the touch-screen buttons. Sometimes I'd accidentally advance too far, lose my place and have to wait for him to come in the evening and help me find my way back.

One little tip in case you ever find yourself unable to see: *Law and Order*. It's the best TV show anyway for someone like me who loves crime procedurals, but it's perfect for the sightless. The characters describe *everything* that is happening, scene by scene:

"What's that?"

"It's a fishing knife. Found it in the corner and it's got blood all over it."

"Well, I've got a blue shirt matching the perp's description. Found it in the clothes hamper at the side of the bed."

"Let's get everything back to the lab for analysis."

Perfect. This must be what radio plays were like. Thank God I wasn't watching the film *Lost in Translation* or something else heavy on visual imagery and short on descriptive dialogue.

Was I scared I'd never see again? Not really. But I'm a stubborn sort and I just assumed this, too, would just take some time to heal and mend itself somehow. Surgery didn't scare me at all—even delicate eye surgery. As long as there was a way out, I just wanted to solve the problem and get on with things.

I was, however, constantly disoriented, which did scare me. I couldn't see the time so hours and days either crawled onward or vanished in a blink of an eye. I couldn't read the aggressive therapy schedule they posted to my wall. They told me a hundred times which one was scheduled and at which time and day, and between the hours of 8 a.m. and 4 p.m., but with my short-term memory problems, it was like a roulette game: I'd hear a knock on my door and wait to hear what was in store for me. Physical therapy with Katie? Occupational therapy? I guess it was kind of nice to constantly be surprised.

One day, a janitor wandered into my room and walked into the shared bathroom. I called out as I heard someone enter, but he didn't answer me. Frightened, I demanded that a sign be posted about my vision and that all guests introduce themselves to me before entering. The nurses didn't need to be asked twice.

As we prepared ourselves for the September eye surgery, the hospital sent a social worker to talk to us about resources for the blind. Finding solutions to work around my vision issues was part of my discharge plan, but I was not ready to be classified as "blind." The suit-and-tie guy was kind, and although he chose his words carefully and focused on offering solutions, I would not listen to anything that required me to contact The Center for the Blind.

"No, I don't need to call them. I won't need special audio computer software. This is temporary. I'm getting surgery. This will go away."

Coughing, he eased into talking about home improvements we might want to make.

Was he *trying* to give me another aneurysm?

Paul immediately escorted him into the hall. He was getting good at sensing my pending emotional explosions.

The kindly suit-and-tie man tried to talk to us once more to deliver the same messages. Paul, in his tactful Scottish way, told the nurses he should never come back. He never did.

PUPPY LOVE

ONE OF THE hardest things about being in the hospital for so long was that I missed my dog, Eddie. I missed his quirky, uneven ears, his sleek black fur and the way he'd energetically wiggle his butt and tail when he was excited. Time would have passed so much faster if I'd had him curled up next to me on the bed, licking my face and demanding attention with those soulful eyes of melted chocolate. Would he remember me when I got home? We'd only had him for about seven months and were still learning how to react to each other.

One day, a solid, wriggling little sandbag of love in the form of an English bulldog plopped onto my bed. A therapy dog! These are dogs whose owners volunteer to bring them to hospitals and nursing homes, cheering up patients and spreading joy. I've heard that pets can do amazing things for people with illnesses, including lowering blood pressure and increasing endorphins just by being there.

This guy was a heavy little lump. But I couldn't stop smiling as I cuddled him and pet his soft fur. I couldn't really see him, but his presence on my bed comforted me and took my mind away from tests, therapy and boredom. It did, however, make me miss Eddie all the more.

And then, surprise! Paul brought Eddie to the hospital to visit me. Our frisky little guy was not allowed inside, but they brought me out to the garden to greet him. I will never forget how it felt to have him jump up into my wheelchair, rest his slim paws on my lap and lick my face. All I wanted to do was hug him and bury my face into his sweet fur and forget about everything that had happened over the last few weeks. I wanted to take him for our usual morning walk along the ship canal, where we could enjoy the sweet-smelling trees, the sounds of coxswains barking at rowers in the early morning mist, and the sight of the Fremont Bridge raising up for passing boats. How long would it be before I could do that with him again? Why couldn't it be right now?

Looking back, I thought I'd be able to get back to our normal routine together in a matter of days. Naiveté can be a friend if you happily forge ahead with no idea how high the mountain is to climb. You just push forward in your ignorance and don't stop to listen to anyone. I wasn't thinking about my sight issues or the overwhelming fatigue I would have to spend months—and even years—fighting. I didn't yet know about the depression, the forgetfulness, the frustration I would face in the times ahead. One step at a time—that's as far into the future as I thought. Even the neuropsychologist who came to assess me expressed some concerns about my "self-appraisal" and thought I might be in a wee bit of denial about my capabilities.

People often ask if a near-death experience changes your outlook. What do you want to do now, they ask? See the pyramids? Travel the world? Bungee jump? I just laugh at all of this. Yes, it does change your outlook in unexpected ways that were revealed to me over my recovery, but you also have very different goals by the end of such a long journey. It becomes more about enjoying the simple pleasures in a more profound way than you did before.

For me, the goal was not to do something crazy, audacious or larger-than-life. It was to get back to normal again. It wasn't about pyramids or thrills or bucket lists. Actually, such big goals just added pressure because they felt so far out of reach at that point in time. All I really longed for was to see again, to walk my dog, to go out to dinner with Paul, to get back to work. My goal was to walk Eddie for thirty minutes every morning. That's it. Simple.

This simple approach helped me avoid becoming overwhelmed, which was one of the biggest effects of the brain injury with which I would consistently struggle. It helped me put one foot in front of the other and make real progress to get back to my life.

SURELY SPAIN WILL CURE WHAT AILS ME

THIS DAMN ANEURYSM had caused upheaval and chaos in our lives. I had very nearly died, but all my doctors pressed upon us how amazing and miraculous my recovery was.

About a year after I recovered, I exchanged some sweet emails with one of my clinical psychologists from rehab:

When I first met you, you were still almost completely blind (as I recall), had a very poor memory, and generally looked like a person who had just survived a very serious SAH. Your recovery has been really remarkable, and I'm not just saying that.

So, yes, I was extremely blessed and lucky in many ways. But at the time, while I was in it, I had absolutely no perspective on what I'd gone through or the recovery that was before me.

During that crazy autumn in the hospital, I faced my first lesson from a teacher that came along and smacked me around quite often during recovery. Patience.

Paul and I had spent early 2008 planning a trip to Northern Spain. Attending a good friend's wedding in Oxford, England kicked off the European vacation, and Paul had splurged by booking us into a posh hotel for that first weekend. Our plan was to then jet off to Bilbao, Spain for a romantic five-day road trip, heading south into the Rioja region to spend the night at a charming winery bodega, then cruising east into the Pyrenees for hiking in the mountains, and finally up to San Sebastian along the northern coast for two days of seaside fun. I also scored us reservations at the Michelin-starred Restaurante Arzak, which was owned by Chef Juan Mari, one of the fathers of modern Basque cuisine, and his daughter Elena. Perfection!

The trip was scheduled for September 10, 2008. About five weeks after all hell broke loose.

Fate played a big role in this entire drama. First, the aneurysm burst while I was at home, not while driving on a busy freeway or stuck in an office surrounded by strangers, which is what I was supposed to be doing that day. Second, my husband decided to come home early the day that I collapsed, which almost certainly saved my life. Follow that with the fact that the region's trauma center was literally a five-minute drive away and the other fact that my hospital network was one of the best in the country for both neurosurgery and rehabilitation, and it was clear that Fate was not only smiling down on me, she was showering me with diamonds.

The way in which I planned our vacation was also somewhat lucky. Normally, I am in charge of trip logistics and keep all the emails and confirmations to myself. But this time, I decided to use a website called TripIt, which meant I could post all of the hotel, flight and dinner information online and share it with Paul.

This made it a snap for him to get in to the itinerary and cancel all of our reservations when the crisis hit.

I, however, was convinced we were still going to get on that plane and fly halfway across the globe. Shaved, blind, frail, weak, underweight, fatigued, cognitively damaged, I still believed we were going to be sunning ourselves in Spain, munching on Manchego and sipping Rioja.

Mind you, Paul told me several times that he had cancelled the trip. But I kept forgetting. I constantly said, "Don't forget to ask the doctor if I can fly with the shunt in my head." Paul would sigh and have to tell me again and again—and watch me get angry again and again.

"But we have to go," I pleaded.

"It'll help me heal," I cajoled.

"We're really not going to be doing much walking. It'll be good for me," I reasoned.

I wasn't even going to be released from the hospital until September 12. But I still thought we were going.

People who didn't know the real me—the medical staff, for instance—thought this was merely my brain injury at play: memory deficiencies, aggression, overemotional outbursts. And it partly was. But I also have an insanely stubborn streak born of my Italian heritage and my status as a feisty redhead. Patience is just not in my vocabulary.

I was forced to learn that life is not on my timeline. This brain injury was one glitch I was not going to be able to overcome with sheer determination and grit. This was serious business and I had serious healing to do. For someone who was used to simply making up her mind and getting things done, how was I going to learn that I could not go from 0 to 100—or hospital bed to Spanish beach—in 60 seconds?

I felt like I'd been punched in the gut the last time Paul told me the trip was cancelled. My brother Michael was in town to help me transition to in-patient rehab and both men were in my room when I again mentioned flying with my shunt.

I could sense Paul's face turning ashen.

"Maria, I told you. There is no Spain. I cancelled the trip."

"What the hell do you mean 'you cancelled the trip'? Why would you do that? I'm fine. I'm going to get discharged soon. I can't believe you did that! "

"I think I'll leave you two alone," said Michael, as he turned on his heel to avoid a repeat of this argument.

"How could you do this?" I burst into tears.

"Maria, you almost *died*. You were on a ventilator. You had a tube in your head. You can't even *see right now!*"

And then I remember saying these exact words to my dear husband, "You need to be my advocate! You're not on my side. I can't believe you let the doctors talk you into this!"

What a freaking brat. I learned later in my rehab groups that frontal lobe damage like mine often results in, among other things, childlike or immature behavior, problems with judgment and impulse control, and unrealistic self-appraisal—both in underestimating as well as overestimating what you can do.[17] But, curiously, none of the literature plainly mentions "brattiness" as an effect.

At one other time in my life, Destiny smacked me full-on in the face to remind me that I could plan things out all I wanted, but God does not work according to my timeline. After nine years of dating and three months to go before our wedding, my college sweetheart and I mutually broke off our engagement. I had always planned to be married with two children by the time I was thirty years old, and it was obviously not going to happen.

Now, once again, I was put in my place when I tried to rally against something I could not control simply by willing it to be so. Most likely this delusion that I can control everything—combined with my inability to surrender to things outside of that control—led to the damn aneurysm in the first place!

I had to learn that this was more serious than I wanted to admit. Several psychologists noted in my chart that they were concerned I didn't fully appreciate the severity of my injury and that I was overestimating my current abilities and recovery time.

Progress had to happen in small steps, not in giant leaps. I was going to have to set some goals yet focus on the immediate step in front of me in order to make any progress. There had already been enough setbacks just while I was in the hospital. And there would be more when I left.

But patience—a virtue with which I've always struggled—finally had me by the throat and I was going to have to listen if I wanted to pick up my life again.

More importantly, I learned during the many months of recovery that having more patience and acceptance didn't mean I wasn't ambitious anymore. Rather, patience was simply something I was going to need more of in my life if I wanted to get off the explosive track I'd been on that had caused the aneurysm in the first place.

It dawned on me that this was the beginning of reframing the way I live my life—if I wanted to have a life to live.

IT TAKES A VILLAGE

IT IS AMAZING how a community rallies when there is a crisis. In the months and years after my brain aneurysm, I was and still am awed by how word spread in Seattle and throughout the country about my condition.

Paul immediately and wisely went into preservation mode when the whole event occurred. He assigned friends or family to act as liaisons who could tell different people in our lives about the situation, as this was the only way for him to keep it together. In order to process what was happening, he focused on a few solid connection points and outsourced the rest. He himself barely knew what was happening from one minute to the next, and I know it must have frustrated many people who care about me not to get real news as it was happening. But we all do what we must to deal with crisis.

For example, as our friend Warren received updates from Paul, his wife Betsy in turn passed on the info to many of our mutual Seattle friends. (I later heard stories from them about where they were when they "got the Maria call.") In some cases, I hadn't known these people for very long, yet my condition had an impact on them. The news seemed to rock people's foundation about the secure lives they all thought they had been leading. "If this can happen to them, it can happen to me," they thought. It's not like I smoke, am obese or abuse drugs, and I'm pretty fit and vivacious. Any excuses they may have made to protect their visions of invincibility did not apply to me—and that left people feeling vulnerable, shaken and wondering how they would react if it had happened to them.

Thank God for social media. Pretty soon, word spread not just via email but via Facebook. People far and wide sent messages to me through the hospital, praying for my speedy recovery. I had visitors constantly throughout the month of August, even though I can't really remember any of them being here. Paul was overwhelmed by the support—so much so, that a few times he had to gently ask well-intentioned friends to please not come to town, not now, not until we knew which way was up.

Another friend remarked months later how she was in awe of the family-like relationships I had built throughout all phases of my life. "You're Italian and have this big, loving, supportive family. And it's like you built another family of friends from every place you've ever lived and every phase of your life. It's inspiring."

Without both of those families, I don't know how I would have recovered.

Becky told Paul about a great website called Caring Bridge, where you can set up a guestbook and blog to centralize communications about a loved one's illness. In late August, they finally set up a page with information on my progress so Paul wouldn't have to keep running up his cell phone bill or typing out emails.

This turned out to be the best emotional gift of all for me. Once it was in place, Paul sat by my bedside and quietly read everyone's guest book posts to me, often three or four times a week. My tears welled up in gratitude. People with whom I had only briefly interacted left messages. People I had worked with years ago and with whom I had lost touch shared their thoughts and good wishes. Newly-made Seattle friends rooted for me.

Such digital support offered powerfully healing mojo, I'll tell you that. It's hard to dwell on your misfortunes when you are so loved and so many people are cheering you on:

"I'm so glad to know you and am grateful for our friendship."
"You are truly a wonder woman.
"I'm sending lots of good energy your way for a full recovery."
"What has happened to you reminds us that life is so fragile and often too short."
"Good job on exceeding expectations. See? Some things haven't changed at all!"

Many people wanted to know what they could do for us. Flowers would have been a waste, since I couldn't see anyway, so Becky coordinated an incidentals fund to cover food, parking, cell phone bills, doggie day care and a host of other little unexpected expenses. After getting home and beginning outpatient rehab, I received a packet from Becky in the mail: a spreadsheet of names and dollar amounts, a check, and pre-addressed thank-you notes since I still couldn't see very well. I wept, not just in gratitude for being alive, but for the boundless generosity in my life.

Believe me; I fully recognize how lucky I am to have such a support network. I can't imagine what people without one would do in this situation. My friends and family gathered around me—physically and virtually—to lift my spirits, which, in my unscientific assessment, accounts for about 80 percent of my recovery.

When I was still in the Neurosurgery Unit, my entourage planned a pizza party to cheer me up. They picked up Serious Pie: *seriously* some of the best thin-crust gourmet pizza in Seattle. While I don't remember this little gathering, I later found out we scarfed everything down and forgot for a little while the seriousness that had brought us all together.

My friend Elizabeth commented in her delightfully sassy way, "This is so good, it's just ridiculous!" and she said that I cracked up at her comment. Here we were, bonding and connecting like my friends and I always have over good food and laughs.

Someone even brought along some beer, and after our party was over, I had leftovers in my little bedside fridge. I would kill to have seen the look on the face of the nurse who cleaned that out after we left.

My visiting friends and family eventually all left Seattle. But they worried about what my prognosis might be. Many were concerned that my eyesight might never return; others wondered if I'd ever get back to my normal self, free of conspiracy theories and memory lapses. No one knew what the lasting brain damage would look like. Almost all of them worried about the strain on Paul, who was forced to be tough but loving during this time. Betsy told me that watching us together was like witnessing a classic love story: Paul held my hand, or spoke softly, or made sure he had all the facts straight from the doctor's most recent instructions. He was very patient with me as I struggled for words or a firm grasp on reality.

Some friends commented that when they came to visit me, I had a hard time remembering who they were but, true to Maria form, I didn't let that stop me from trying to chat. I asked questions and tested my memory of them as we talked. Paul gently reminded me if I was wrong, as it was important to my recovery to know when I was inaccurately remembering something.

To support Paul, Warren and Betsy contacted their friend Karen, a personal chef, to see what she'd charge to cook for Paul and all the out of town guests staying with us. Warren started a donation fund among Microsoft colleagues who were eager to help. Everyone ate very well for an entire month while I lay in the hospital enjoying my own surprisingly delicious omelets, pancakes and chocolate cake.

In a way, this whole brain aneurysm thing was like having the chance to attend my own funeral. I know that sounds morbid but hear me out. I got to see just how much I meant to everyone in my life. Even today, a lump still catches in my throat when I think about those people who rearranged their lives and came to Seattle. *For me.* And all of those who reached out via email or phone to offer support: people I assumed had forgotten me from two jobs ago, or those I only interacted with briefly, such as theatre co-stars and volunteer project partners—they all showed up. They all shared a prayer, an encouragement, a hilarious memory or a "You go, girl!" I think this propped up not only me, but my poor, exhausted Paul as well.

I have struggled my entire life with yearning to make a real impact on people's lives, to give back, and to offer inspiration and support. And I always thought I fell short in so many ways. I'm pretty hard on myself and if I'm not literally saving lives in Africa, I'm not sure what value I'm adding to this planet. Maybe this entire journey was God's way of slapping me in the face and saying, "Quit sulking! You *do* impact people; you *do* make a difference in their lives! Look, see?"

I am humble enough to recognize that seeing this ordeal as a gift is a luxury. It's only due to my amazing recovery that I can look back and appreciate it all. I'm not on medication for the rest of my life, or relying on a walker, or unable to communicate my words clearly. I know that. I saw such devastation during my rehab group therapies. So I know it's a bit arrogant to say this was all a gift. But, honestly, it was.

God showed me that, no matter what, you need to count on your tribe for support when times get tough. You don't always have to be strong, or brave or even independent. People often can and do show the most glorious versions of themselves during a crisis.

But the hospital stay was just the beginning of the journey, and there were many challenges, still unknown to us at the time, we would face. Recovery out in the real world soon proved to me just how much I needed to count on my tribe if I was ever going to get my life back again.

ALTERED GOALS

IN THE BEGINNING of 2008, I set a list of goals for the year. I had clearly seen myself as Maria Ross: Woman with a Mission.

Start and build my business and personal brand into a powerhouse of marketing, writing and acting.

Act. Continue acting and break into the Seattle theatre community with work on some shows or acting classes.

Write. Commit to writing through my blog, my novel idea and other articles like my wine column once a month.

Build wealth. Continue to build our financial independence through savings and investment. Build a budget and live within our means as we have been.

Stay healthy. Commit to health and balance with yoga two to three times a week, and find a cardio program (spinning, walking, belly dancing) I enjoy two times a week. Walk 30 minutes every day.

Get inspired. Read Eleanor Roosevelt's biography. Read On Writing.

Give back to the world. Find some causes to rally behind with my time and my money.

Be an open, loving, listening and supportive wife, friend, daughter and sister.

Get a dog.

Live with gratitude. Appreciate the life and blessings I have RIGHT NOW.

I was well on my way to achieving most of them when this unexpected crisis struck. I soon had a whole team of people helping me set new goals, but not in the way I had planned.

While at the hospital, we met several times with our care team. During these checkpoints, we set goals, asked questions, and met with the doctors, therapists and others involved in my daily care. The meetings gave Paul an opportunity to confer with medical staff he may have missed on rounds or those who were not available during his visits.

Although my memory issues gave me trouble, these meetings made me feel that I had a say in my own destiny. And at a time when most of your dignity is completely stripped away, these meetings—and getting to choose my own food at each meal—helped me start the long process toward taking care of myself again.

One of our meetings was dedicated to setting my discharge goals. At first, they couldn't really give me a discharge date, as they were monitoring progress and also trying to see what my rehab needs would be. But we set some goals that, once attained, would be a good indicator that I was ready to rock and roll.

Recently, I found my list of these discharge goals tucked away in a file. When I read them, I wept. These were my lofty goals—post-aneurysm—in the fall of 2008:

At the time of discharge, I will be able to:
Get myself dressed and obtain my clothes by myself
Go to and from the bathroom by myself
Complete a shower by myself
Explore options for reading and computer access
Walk outdoors with someone nearby
Go up and down three flights of stairs by myself
Do twenty minutes of cardio exercises without a rest
Do a strengthening program daily on my own

What a different list than the one which began 2008. Yet when we set these goals, they seemed so ambitious. I was excited when I got approved to leave the hospital after having met all of these goals.

Now when I read these goals and compare them to what I'd been planning earlier in the year, I feel like someone punched me in the gut—hard.

Shortly before my hospital discharge, I was evaluated by Rehab Without Walls, an in-home rehab care company. Part of UWMC's discharge procedure is to ensure the patient has ample support and structure to continue healing at home. The staff felt this would be an excellent option for me to continue making progress in my recovery. Based on my frail state and the as yet unknown full extent of my brain damage, it was clear to everyone that I had a long road back to health and independence.

Just reading the recommendations that Rehab Without Walls made in their evaluation report exhausts me today. At the time, Paul must have felt pretty overwhelmed reading everything I was going to need. When you start out on a long journey, sometimes the sheer magnitude of what you're in for can paralyze you:

Maria had made gains during her hospitalization but still needs intensive rehab services to continue making these gains and to maximize her independence.

Maria will need physical therapy to assist with improving her strength and endurance and with becoming independent with household mobility due to her limited vision.

She needs continued work with ambulation outside and with her dog.

She needs occupational therapy to assist with becoming independent on all of her basic ADLs (Activities of Daily Living) and to begin working on her higher level ADLs, including cooking, laundry and caring for her dog.

She needs speech therapy to assist with learning compensatory strategies for her short-term memory, cognitive deficits and visual impairments.

She will need psychosocial counseling services to assist her with coping and adjustment issues.

She will need rehab specialists to assist the therapists in running the programs written for her, as well as to evaluate Maria's ability to be left alone safely.

Good God that is one daunting list of needs.

PART THREE

Life Rebooted

*Take the first step in faith. You don't have to see the whole staircase,
just take the first step.*

- Martin Luther King, Jr.

*Start by doing what's necessary; then do what's possible; and suddenly
you are doing the impossible.*

- St. Francis of Assisi

GOING HOME

AN ORDERLY WHEELED me to our waiting car in the hospital loading zone. I couldn't get in fast enough. Going home at last!

It was September 12, 2008. More than five weeks after our ordeal had begun.

Riding in the car was an odd sensation, with the wind on my face from the open window. While it was incredibly freeing, I felt like I was on a trapeze, high above the ground, and without a net.

Leaving the safe confines of the hospital for the wider world left me vulnerable and uncertain. Were things going to feel immediately normal again upon stepping into our house? What would I do on this first day? The rules had changed and it dawned on me that I had no idea how to handle this first day and night on our own.

I'm not sure what I imagined during that ride home. Maybe I fooled myself into thinking I was going to dive right back into work again. I had been telling my doctors and therapists I planned to get back to work in December. Arms folded and eyes doubtful, I could sense their disbelief.

"Poor girl," I could hear them thinking. "She is totally deluding herself."

But really, I thought, it couldn't take that long, could it?

I had cleared all of my discharge goals to some degree. Walking outdoors still required some assistance due to my eyesight. With in-home speech therapy and some additional psych testing, I continued to explore options for memory strategies. I could climb the stairs and maintain balance using a cane (which Paul and I affectionately termed The Whacking Stick, because I looked like a crazy old woman when I playfully shook it at him) and it also helped me ensure I was clear of all obstacles when walking. My legs were still weak and the cane gave me something to lean on when fatigued.

My discharge sheet advised that I could only be up and about unassisted in known environments that were free of obstacles, and that I could only be in unknown territory when I had assistance from family or friends. It also instructed "NO DRIVING" (written in all caps) and no lifting of anything greater than 10 pounds.

Part-time assistance came in the form of friends and hired health aides. Paul had to go to work and it just wasn't safe to leave me alone in the house because of my sight and memory issues. I had mastered carefully taking a shower on my own—and amazingly enough, shaving my legs again (being brain injured is no excuse for stubble!)—by feeling my way around but still required someone to be nearby just in case I fell. Or sliced my leg open.

My left eye surgery, a vitrectomy, was slated for September 19. One week away. Surely, I thought, I can manage things by myself for a week without babysitters and then everything will be fine.

Ha.

We opened the door and I was immediately greeted by Eddie bounding down the stairs. Oh, it was so nice to be with him again! Paul settled me onto the couch and I think we then tried to figure out what to have for lunch. It was moment to moment, both of us fumbling for what to do next.

The home health aides did not arrive until Monday, when Paul went to work. That weekend is not ingrained in my memory too well, but to hazard a guess, I probably slept and "watched" TV most of the time.

Monday rolled around and a soft-spoken, fifty-something former flower child whom I'll call Sally came to our door. Paul delayed his leaving with various excuses and, finally, with my promise that we'd be okay, he left us.

It was a bit like being under a microscope or having your house bugged with a webcam. Part of me wanted to be a hostess and entertain this guest, but part of me realized I needed to just do whatever I was going to do. Sally helped me with my shower that morning and then sat at the table reading books while I lounged and listened to the TV. Woo hoo. Excitement galore. To pass time, she also did some household chores, which was pretty awesome. She helped prepare lunch for me and even took Eddie out during the day.

For as nice as she was, it was one of the most excruciatingly long days of my life. I wasn't sure what to do around her. She eased my mind a bit when she said, in her motherly tone of voice, "I'm used to this. You can sleep or watch TV or do whatever you need to do. Don't worry about me, I'm just fine!"

One thing I will never forget about Sally: the apples. Behind our townhome is a residential access alley and across the alley stands a medium-sized apple tree. In the fall, ripe apples drop all over the little patch of open lawn. Sally asked me about them and if it was okay to take some.

"I like to bake apple pies," she said.

Of course she did. I wouldn't have been surprised if she knitted and baked cookies as well. She was so damn cute! I told her no one ever collects those apples, so she could go for it. A few days later, she told me how delicious the pies had turned out. Funny, the things we choose to remember about people.

Sally stayed with me a few days a week. My friend Barb came to pinch-hit a few times, and then I had another woman—an Eastern European nursing student—for one day a week. She talked even less than Sally and, since she was younger, I felt even more uncomfortable with her there, watching my every move.

Their responsibilities were not just to care for me, give me my medications or ensure I didn't fall, but to also help with light housekeeping and lunch prep. The aides had a binder and recorded everything—and I mean everything—that I did each day:

Maria took a shower and dressed herself. I stood by for assist.

Maria is a very pleasant person to work with. Today, she had a bowl of cereal and blueberries for breakfast. I made her a peanut butter and jelly sandwich for lunch and then wiped down the counters and appliances.

Maria went out for a walk with the physical therapist. I folded laundry. She then took a short nap.

Maria has another busy day of therapy today. Rehab is coming at 11:30 a.m. and her speech therapist is coming at 2:00 p.m.

Maria always has a smile on her face.

Relief from the awkwardness often came when my home therapists came by for sessions. Rehab Without Walls dispatched physical, occupational and speech therapists to my house a few days a week. This way, I could continue my regimen of strength-building and cognitive assistance.

I started toward my goal of walking Eddie for thirty minutes in the PT sessions. We leashed him up, and then I wrapped my arm around the therapist's arm, very tightly, and off we went. At first, we made it halfway around the block. That left me needing a two-hour nap. But over time we built up to the entire block, and eventually, to the start of the ship canal trail (a few blocks from our house) and back. Thirty minutes was still a long way away but we were making progress.

In addition, our house never looked as clean and tidy as when those home health aides were with us. Dare I even say I could have found a way to get used to that?

ONE-EYED WILLIE

SEPTEMBER 19, 2008. Finally, *finally*, I would be able to see a bit better. The day for my vitrectomy surgery in my left eye was upon us. Oh joy! I couldn't wait to get past this whole vision problem and just get on with my life.

Paul drove me back to the hospital we had left just a week before, and I was prepped for surgery. I really didn't want to know too many details about what the surgeon was going to do, because anything involving poking eyeballs makes me squeamish and sends me into shivers. The medical team was going to put me under, do its thing, and then—poof—I'd wake up with sight in my left eye. That's all I needed to know.

In the recovery unit, I surfaced into consciousness and felt a stabbing in my left eye that intensified as I came to. I have never, before or since, felt that type of raw, screeching pain in my life. Such pain is not typical with this procedure but because of my small frame, the nurses carefully administered a more conservative dose of pain killers. I begged for more morphine.

Paul was right there as I cried in agony, squeezing his hand. He pleaded with the nurse, "Please give her more drugs!"

"But she's so little!" said the poor nurse. "I'm giving her as much as I can!"

Vomiting is a part of coming out of anesthesia. Combine that with intense pain, and you get even more nauseous. I kept throwing up, hiccupping back sobs of pain, and throwing up again. It was awful. My eye was bandaged so I couldn't even see if this pain was worth it.

But it was! When things calmed down and I came to again, the pain was still simmering but much less intense. The doctor came in to remove the bandage and check things out. As he peeled away the layer, I held my breath.

He shined a bright light at my left eye, and I looked up and finally saw the face of Dr. Kinyoun for the first time. I cried out with joy when I saw his silver hair and mischievous grin. From his voice, I had pictured the actor who plays Roger on *Mad Men*: a tall, sophisticated and dapper older gentleman. I wasn't too far off—although Dr. Kinyoun is a bit shorter.

Sending me home with various medicinal eye drops, the doctor scheduled several follow-up visits with me. Over the course of the next eight months, I visited Dr. Kinyoun every four to six weeks so he could track my progress.

Having sight again was wonderful and a luxury I never again took for granted. The new challenge was to get used to seeing out of only one eye for a while. My depth perception was totally screwed up. My right eye was still full of gunk, as I liked to call it, and was of no real use to me. It's a lot harder to handle one eye than you'd think!

"How did pirates manage this?" I joked with Paul.

Because of this, I still needed help getting around, as my confidence was shot just as much as my sight was impaired. Curbs and stairs were a challenge due to the depth perception issues, and I had increased night-blindness issues, so I was not very good in the dark. Low lighting also became a general problem for "one-eyed Maria," because I couldn't make out the outlines of obstacles very well. I grabbed onto the railing and tapped my toe forward until I felt the drop of a stair and knew I could continue.

At least now I could begin my physical, cognitive and occupational therapies in earnest. I would be able to take the cognitive and neuropsychology tests needed to assess just how much brain damage I had suffered. I could see out of one eye and all indications were that my vision would improve over time, but was I really ready for those tougher answers?

PERSONAL TRAINING: BRAIN INJURY STYLE

THE PHYSICAL THERAPIST, occupational therapist, and speech therapist who came to my home had their own unique goals for me, but they all had one underlying question to answer: does Maria understand what she is doing?

I needed to "demonstrate the ability to independently evacuate in an emergency situation to reduce supervision requirements." This meant that I had to verbalize if various emergencies were worthy of calling 9-1-1 or not. Some of them included:

There is a fire in the kitchen
Someone is breaking into the back door
The mail has not been delivered (my personal fave...can you imagine
    calling the police on that one?)
I fell, got back into the chair and am now okay
There is a fire in the garage
There is a loud noise coming from the washer
We are out of peanut butter (another classic!)

I found it both humorous and poignant to note that in my life I've had intelligent political debates, passionate conversations about faith, and lively critiques about the message an independent film director is really trying to convey and yet I was brought so low as to question my mental ability to cope with running out of Skippy Peanut Butter.

Yet this became my new reality during recovery.

I tried to think of it as having my own personal trainer come to my house and whip me into shape. Granted, the weights were at most one pound each, and the exercises consisted mostly of stretches or pulling a light band up, down and across my body. The goal was to increase my balance and decrease the risk of falls. I also wanted to increase my strength and endurance to "allow for functional mobility and increased independence for Activities of Daily Living." I laughed with my PT as I regaled her with tales of how I used to kick ass in spin class. But when you get winded going up the two flights of stairs in your own home, you really just gotta start somewhere.

The occupational therapist was helpful in making sure I could do things for myself in my home setting, especially when I used knives to prepare food. I flushed with victory when she handed me a red bell pepper and a knife—a real one with sharp edges—and I chopped my enemy into chunks on the cutting board. When I turned to her in triumph, her hand was up and ready to meet mine in a high five.

"Passed!" she said.

The one person I really struggled with was my speech therapist. In the beginning, I didn't fully appreciate the severity of what had happened to me. I knew that memory was an issue but really didn't grasp that everyone was still unsure as to my cognitive damage. Just as I had in the hospital, I got impatient with her as she tested me on simple things that I felt I easily could handle, like defining very basic words, filling in sentences from a multiple-choice group of words, or detecting patterns in number sequences. Yet unbeknownst to me, she really was testing deeper skills to see how much my frontal lobe had been impacted.

The pressure from the initial aneurysm bleed in my brain had triggered the vasospasm that snapped my blood vessels shut, causing a lack of blood flow for a bit into my frontal lobe. This restriction is also called *ischemia*, which can result in tissue damage or dysfunction. Basically, some of my brain cells started to die.

If your brain were a fighter jet, the frontal lobe would be the well-trained pilot who manages all the instruments and settings. The frontal lobe controls many of the so-called executive skills that I count on to make my living: organization, decision-making, multi-tasking, and prioritization are a few examples. The frontal lobe also regulates impulse control and damage to that area can cause personality changes, such as becoming more irritable or aggressive.

While I was in the hospital, a young, bespectacled rehab psychologist named Dr. Ivan Molton visited me. He's trained to screen brain injury patients for depression and anxiety—partially to ensure patients are not suicidal but also to help with cognitive rehabilitation and coping skills for memory, attention, and language challenges. Many people don't get all their functions back, but his job is to help them find creative ways to adapt.

When Dr. Molton first met me, I was blind, shorn and frail. His notes of that first visit state:

Patient reports ongoing trouble with her memory in complex environments. Pleasant, cooperative woman with a subarachnoid hemorrhage and visual and cognitive impairment. She is denying significant problems with mood, pain, anxiety and sleep and is motivated to engage in rehab therapies. She demonstrates moderate insight into the nature of her cognitive deficits, although she appears to be aware of the severity of memory disruption. She is appropriately distressed about her vision loss, although she believes this change to be mostly temporary. Adjustment may be an issue for her down the road when the nature and severity of her cognitive deficits interacts with the demands of her work.

Later, he told me "moderate" in his shorthand means he had concerns that I didn't fully appreciate the extent of my injury or my length of recovery. I couldn't agree more.

I think this was why the speech therapy was so frustrating to me. I had not yet learned all I would learn about what was going on in my brain. Since I felt fine, could speak, could recognize people, and could read and comprehend, I thought this whole "getting back to my life" thing would be a piece of cake. Physically, I knew I needed work. But that was much more tangible. How do you tell someone they are not as good at "prioritizing" until they actually need to prioritize?

This is a common problem with the way our society views brain injury. That football player who just got slammed in the head may be able to tell you his name and the date and shake it off, but you have no idea what the long-term effects are to his cognitive stability. "You look fine," is not a medical diagnosis when it comes to the brain. Brain injury can be an unseen disability—if you want to use that word—with lasting impacts that often only the patient can see and recognize.

I could tell that my memory was impacted. That was a given. And I did start to notice that where once I used to come up with just the right snarky, quick-witted remark, I was struggling for the right words. Vocabulary had always been a strong suit of mine, as shown when my brothers, six years older than me and in high school, would occasionally consult me on proper spelling. But I could tell words were not as readily available as they used to be. Sometimes I'd struggle to come up with the right word, like "appointment" or "café," when I was talking with someone. I'd always been a fan of witty banter, but conversations were a little hard to keep up with and sly comebacks did not pop to mind quite as fast as they had. I processed what was being said and thought about my reply, but by then the discussion had moved on.

I'm just out of practice, I thought. I need to get my edge back.

I was still in the denial phase that accompanies any change in life. But I didn't have concrete proof until later.

Besides, I had other things to deal with. I filled my days with naps, therapy and sometimes visits with friends. I tried getting back into my morning ritual of eating breakfast at our kitchen counter, reading my Wall Street Journal (with a magnifying glass now) and taking Eddie for his walk.

My home therapies were completed by mid-October. After about four weeks, I passed all the tests and met all the objectives of rehab. Now I just needed to take responsibility for my own exercise regime while healing. I had dozens of follow-up doctor visits for various things and I even tried to do some light yoga at home with a DVD and a friend—of course, I couldn't really do a full downward dog yet because it still felt tender to invert my head.

Paul also purchased Wii Fit and I made a game of practicing my balance and coordination skills. Wii Fit has players weigh themselves at the beginning of each fitness session. My little avatar (the cartoon image of me that popped up on-screen) usually swooned, and Wii told me in its chirpy little voice, "You are underweight."

Really? Thanks for the update.

My doctors could not believe my rapid recovery, which probably kept me in denial even longer about any long-term effects. As Paul wrote in the online Caring Bridge journal, *Looking back six weeks, we did not expect for Maria to be home, watching* Law and Order *reruns and using Wii Fit. We are very lucky.*

But I soon learned about the surprising and ugly side of brain injury.

Emotionally and psychologically, I was struggling. As Paul went back to a regular work schedule, I started to feel anxious and panicky when he wasn't around. Every day I'd watch the clock until he got home from work. To kill time, I'd nap or play with Eddie...thinking twenty minutes had passed, I was sorely disappointed to realize it had only been five. Together, Paul and I ventured out to a few restaurants and outings with friends, but I very quickly wanted to get back into the comfort zone of my house.

Friends took great care of me. They chauffeured me places and ensured I had an arm to grab onto when tackling stairs or walking over curbs in the dark. They complimented my short hair as it grew in, and my book club even selected titles that I could get as audio books, because reading print still strained my eyes if I did it for long periods of time.

Unfortunately, I felt myself turning into a bit of a recluse. It was so much effort to gear up for seeing someone, and I was left drained and exhausted. I just wanted to sit on the couch with Eddie and watch TV all day. I was literally afraid to leave the house, as if I was tethered to an oxygen tank and if I went too far, I wouldn't be able to breathe.

My excuse was that I was in recovery and healing. It didn't alleviate the guilt I felt about lying around all day, but it was enough to rationalize my behavior. And it's not like I got a whole heck of a lot done inside the house either: I couldn't even motivate myself to do one load of laundry.

Paul tried to help me though this, even though he didn't understand what was happening either. I couldn't face a to-do list, so he said, "Why not just make one goal for the day?"

He was literally doing everything: working, cleaning, cooking, driving. He really needed some help.

So, with all good intentions, I kept promising, "I'll do the laundry today." Or, "I'll clean the bathroom." And the day slipped away without it getting done.

I didn't understand what was happening. It was like someone sucked all my "get up and go" out of me. I had a goal, I had a plan; I just couldn't move. Such excuses as "I'll just watch one more show" or "I'll wait until after lunch" became like football sideline chains I could move down the field in avoidance. For someone used to juggling work, acting, volunteering, networking and running here, there and everywhere as people marveled, "Where the hell do you find the time?" this was clearly not right. I cried most days in frustration and bewilderment at what was happening to me.

Paul was understanding but he eventually got to a breaking point—not about my failure to do chores, but about my utter lack of initiation or steam. He didn't know what to do for me. I could hear it in his clipped tone as he struggled to hide his bottled-up frustration, and I could see it in his pleading eyes as he tried one approach after another.

Yet because I was like a raw emotional nerve, even talking about it brought me to tears. The stress of not knowing what to do was too much to bear and it strained our relationship. I could tell he often bit his tongue because, after all, I was the patient. We were caught in this weird limbo of being out of immediate danger but not being back to "normal" yet either. How the hell was I going to get back to the way I was? And *when*?

Soon, some light cut through the fog of our darkness as we learned more about what we were facing.

NEVER MET A TEST I DIDN'T LIKE . . . UNTIL NOW

M Y FRIENDS AND family must have had clandestine hallway conversations out of my earshot, saying things like, "She's smoking crack if she thinks she won't need help," especially after they heard some of my crazy answers to simple tests I was often given in the hospital.

The hospital psychologists felt that, although I performed above expected levels in verbal learning, memory, and attention, my reasoning fell below expected levels and my judgment was "in the severely impaired range for function." Another report stated:

> *This is consistent with reports from the treatment team who state, for example, that Maria has stated that she will not need anyone with her once she gets home (despite new blindness) and that even with her vision difficulties, she will need her husband to go only once with her before she is able to walk the dog on her own.*

But they also stated I was positive, friendly and cooperative, and had a good sense of humor. So the real Maria was still inside of me, yearning to get out.

The doctors requested a neuropsychological evaluation eight to ten weeks after my discharge to evaluate cognitive improvements and red-flag any problem areas. Basically, it was a "sanity check" to make sure I understood the full extent of any difficulties and to put together a plan to deal with them before returning to full-time work. A day-long marathon testing session was scheduled for November 2008.

I was intrigued and nervous about this test. As I understood it, there would be a series of tests, challenges, puzzles and questions similar to those on a college entrance exam. An honors student, I have always reveled in tests and rankings. Paul jokes that I crave measurement to constantly see where I stack up against others and if I've earned bragging rights. I take a slightly more positive view: I am a sucker for feedback and always want to know how I can improve, advance and up my game. Self-assessments, critiques, performance reviews, report cards...I love them all. And yes, I'm a tad competitive. I guess that's why I love useless trivia games so much: I'm pretty damn good at them.

I shared this little fact about being a *Jeopardy* addict when I went in for testing and even hinted that I was not quite as quick on my answers as I used to be. Little did I know the test actually began the moment I walked in the door and even my polite small talk with the testing administrator was noted in my results report. Yikes.

The day consisted of so many different tests, I can't remember them all. They measured me on vocabulary, arithmetic, comprehension, reasoning, picture arrangements, memory, spatial relationships, motor skills—you name it.

It was like a giant, day-long game show with various challenges and puzzles to solve. (I can't describe in too much detail the tests I remember taking that day. Putting such information out in the public domain could alter test results for future patients if they know what to expect. This might mask subtle problems they are having and could skew results and recommendations. Suffice it to say I got to play word games, number games, pattern games and even games of observation and recall.)

One test had me look inside a very 1970s slide machine viewer and note different patterns and shapes as they flashed in front of me. Other tests assessed my visual spatial and tactual spatial problem solving. Basically, solving challenges while I was able to see what I was doing versus only performing the task by touch. For example, I had a board with cutouts and was given various wooden shapes to place into their respective openings. The test administrators found I had mild impairment when I tried to "integrate the efforts of both hands." The theory was that "it is possible for anterior communicating artery aneurysms to disrupt inter-hemisphere communication so that problem-solving attempts involving both hands working together are not as efficient as problem-solving using one hand alone."

Hmm. Who knew?

They saw mild inefficiency with my left hand as opposed to my right and "mild inattention to the left side of space." I seemed to not get as many of the shapes placed as quickly or accurately on the left side of the board versus the right side. They chalked that up to the aneurysm impacting the right side of my brain, which controls the left side of your body.

As the day dragged on, I was forced to do math in my head (never a strong suit for me anyway), although I was pleased to score in the 84th percentile on that, which they deemed "excellent."

The one test that really frustrated me was word lists. The test administrator gave me a list of about twelve unrelated pairs of words (e.g., "cargo" and "pecan") and then I'd be tested on recalling all of the pairs—in order.

Are you freaking kidding me? Who the hell is good at this when you can't even associate the two words in your head? And there seemed to be *so* many pairs to remember.

They tested stuff like this a few times to check both recent and then delayed memory. I got snippy with the tester on this one.

"But this makes no sense! None of these words are even remotely related. I would have had to write them down before the aneurysm, too. How can you test memory on something that is difficult for even a normal person to remember?"

The math ones also really upset me. I mean, some of this stuff was *hard*, like long-forgotten formulas and algorithms from calculus or algebra. I went to college and (from what they told me) scored very high on my IQ test. But what about someone not as lucky or educated as me? I did not know at the time that these tests are normed and graded by education level so everyone has a level playing field.

"What about people who don't even have a high school education?" I protested. "This test would be totally unfair to them!"

Yep, they noted this "outburst" on my chart as well:

There was also some irritability present during testing that is quite uncharacteristic for most individuals with Maria's professional and educational background otherwise and may reflect some very mild decrease in affect regulation. Even in the context of reports of premorbid personality tendencies to be somewhat impatient and irritable at times.

"Decrease in affect regulation"—my eye! Just talk to managers or co-workers I've had. I've never been afraid to say what I really think. Especially since I don't have a poker face. I used to have a boss who could just read my anger, confusion, or total disagreement without me uttering a word. "What is that face, Maria?" she'd tease.

I had told the doctors I had a short fuse before this whole incident and that now it was just non-existent. Hence the "even in the context of reports of premorbid personality tendencies." Sheesh.

Apparently, the test was assessing my reactions and mood, and not just my performance, to see what types of personality changes I might have. How was I handling the pressure? How was I problem solving?

I'm not sure any other type of bodily injury can have quite the same impact on who you are as a person as a brain injury can. I mean, your personality defines who you are, no matter what you are physically capable of. If that gets altered in any way, are you really who you were? Or is your identity something deeper, in your soul? Aren't we really just the sum of the personality traits we act on and the feelings that we have?

For example, if you were a very passive, meek person and yet, after a brain injury, you become violent and aggressive, is that who you are? If a brain injury can alter that—beyond anything physical—then who are we?

If my ability to articulate my viewpoint really well, or sling a quick-witted comeback during happy hour, or craft a detailed project plan was changed forever, then how do I define myself? Can I still claim to be a type A perfectionist? Can I still boast of being detail-oriented or good with names? I'm not sure.

It's kind of weird when you think about this, but do the mechanics of our brain as an organ define who we are? Guess it depends on how you view your innate self and how it is formed. If you really believe that who you are is deep, soulful and spiritual, then how can a brain injury take that away?

Yet it seems to do so quite often, from everything I've seen and read.

So what was that going to mean for me?

After this exhausting day of tests, the conclusion was that I performed "remarkably well across a wide range of tasks, especially given the recency and severity of her stroke." Other than some of the left side issues, the report stated that I had mild to moderate difficulty with my executive functions: things like planning, organizing, and strategy development. The report also pointed out that I had some issues with inference and implication, meaning I was interpreting analogies way too literally. I also had some "word generation" issues, such as when they flashed up pictures and asked me to quickly come up with the name of each item.

I had trouble discerning important details from non-important ones. This filtering problem (which is common to many frontal lobe brain injuries) turned out to be at the root of many challenges down the road.

The test results indicated that I should continue speech therapy to assist with executive function, efficient verbal explanation and complex verbal memory retrieval, as well as strategy development (i.e., finding ways to adapt and work around my deficits). My ability to acquire, retain and retrieve complex verbal information could be problematic, they said, in the context of being self-employed. They recommended I gradually return to work so I could trial any new tricks and techniques for overcoming my issues. Plus, I was also going to need lots of rest as I battled fatigue and exerted new efforts on what had been routine and automatic for me before the injury.

The doctors felt that templates, procedures and checklists would be helpful aids so I could keep track of clients, work, and conversations. They also suggested my first trial projects back on the job be well-structured and scoped; sort of like training wheels as I got my mojo back. I did not heed this advice very well.

But overall, I had done well.

"In my twenty-five years of practice, I've never seen someone perform as well as you did on this test, given the severity of your injury," said the lead psychologist. She said I had a few "hitches in my giddy'up" that I needed to work on but other than that, I had done extremely well for someone who'd lived through what I'd lived through. Once again, I was struck with how lucky I was to have dodged a bullet.

And at least now, my cognitive issues had names and I was aware they existed. Know thy enemy, they always say. Articulating my issues was the first step to conquering them.

I breathed a sigh of relief.

Later, I wrestled with where that left me as a person and how I defined myself. Farther down the road, I found out that the emotional and psychological effects of my frontal lobe brain damage were going to be bigger adversaries than anything related to word lists or wooden shapes.

THE NECKLACE

MY HAIR WAS shaved off, I couldn't see, I hadn't worn makeup in over two months and who knows what my wayward brows must have looked like. The gal who adored getting a mani/pedi every few weeks and wearing cute, strappy sandals was nowhere to be seen. I was in PJs or jeans and T-shirts almost every day. Having lost over 20 pounds off my already petite frame, I resembled a prisoner of war. One of my first nights home from the hospital, Paul gasped and choked back tears when he saw me dressing for bed.

"You're so thin!"

Something every wife loves to hear, to be sure, but not in that pained tone of voice.

Vanity, thy name is woman. How idiotic is it that I didn't feel like myself because I wasn't able to accessorize? I'm not an overly high-maintenance fashionista; I love donning ripped jeans and a baseball hat on occasion and will not cancel a lunch date just because I forgot to apply mascara. That would be crazy.

But despite all of the cognitive and psychological changes I was experiencing, nothing starkly contrasted the old me and the new me more than my physical appearance.

I felt like a patient: frail, pale and ghostly. The lack of make-up and dressing up hammered that point home to me during those early recovery days. I was not Maria; I was a brain injury survivor. I was someone who needed caregivers and therapists. I was no longer the attractive, vivacious, style-conscious person my husband had married. I felt homely, androgynous, and sick.

Thinking this way then led to feeling vain and ungrateful, so I often experienced a double whammy of ickiness.

Don't lynch me. I recognized, even at the time, that I was lucky to be alive and I had to give myself time to heal before worrying about whether I was wearing the right length jeans for those sexy high heels. No one talks about this part of surviving trauma or recovering from illness because I think we feel so badly for admitting it. My adorable girlfriends had purchased a pair of tweezers for me while I was in the hospital, along with some scented lotion and facial cleanser to at least help me feel a bit more normal. At one point, I even think Paul unsteadily tweezed my brows when I asked him.

As women, the ugly truth is that we often do feel confident and on top of the world when we look attractive and pulled together, and I was none of those things right now. It was just another cue that I was not back in the groove of my life yet; another reminder that I had a long way to go, no matter how much I tried to deny it or power on through.

After being home a few weeks, a small package arrived. Tearing it open, I found a box and a handwritten note from a fabulous jewelry designer friend in LA, Nancy Dobbs-Owen. She and I had met years ago through Becky and she designed and crafted all my wedding jewelry for me and my bridesmaids. I love her work: she artfully wires together brilliant crystals and stones into "flowers" that adorn necklaces, bracelets and earrings. Her note wished me well and said she was thinking of me every day since she'd heard the news. She was sending this gift along to cheer me up during my recovery and she hoped it brought a smile to my face.

Inside was a gorgeous triple-strand golden choker and at its center rested a flower shape with petals made of pearlescent peachy-white stones.

Still in yoga pants and a T-shirt, I immediately tried it on. It transformed me. The Old Me seemed to hang around my neck and brighten my face, telling me I was not so far gone after all. Beautiful celebrities were sporting Nancy's jewelry and so was I. I could still shine.

That necklace gave me hope that I still had the old Maria in me and that I would see her again someday.

I wore that necklace to almost every outing over the next few months.

GIVING THANKS FOR . . . EMERGENCY SURGERY?

"WELL, YOUR LEFT retina is detaching and we'll need to operate as soon as possible. When are you free next week?"

Screech. What? Huh...? This was just a routine check-in with Dr. Kinyoun. By now I was used to the standard drill: chat with the technician, eye pressure check and eye chart test, dilation drops and a thorough routine of eye gymnastics with the doctor. He'd have me look up, down, to the right and to the left and then he shined the brightest light this side of Broadway into my eyes, until they involuntarily rolled back in my head. I had been enjoying the upward trend of my recovery when it all came to a screeching halt.

"That can't be. I'm flying home for Thanksgiving next week," I sputtered. As if that would miraculously force my eye to heal itself.

"One of the risks of the eye surgery you had, especially with your pre-existing condition of lattice degeneration, was that your retina might detach," Dr. Kinyoun told me. "Our eyes are sensitive and just don't like being messed around with, so a surgery like you had can often result in something like this. When can you come in?"

"But you don't understand. I have to go home. We leave tomorrow. You just found this. Can't it wait just a week and be done when I get back?"

Dr. Kinyoun thought about this for a moment. It was not ideal. A detached retina, once it starts, can degrade in a very short period of time.

My family had been an amazing support for us during this difficult time. They flew in at a moment's notice to be by my side and constantly checking in with me during my recovery. I know the ordeal was especially hard on my older parents, both about eighty, as they had their own physical issues to deal with while worrying about me. In a way, I felt guilty for putting them through all of that, even though I fully know it was not my fault. I mean, really, who would choose a brain hemorrhage?

Paul and I vowed to make it home to Columbus, Ohio for Thanksgiving. It felt more important to gather our family together than it ever had before. This was my first travel since the brain injury. With my current anxious state and the difficult time I was having at being overwhelmed by too much activity, inputs, lights, sounds and people, the trip was going to be a particular challenge: buzzing airport, a thousand little tasks to complete when packing, being in any environment other than my home, and of course my boisterous, lively, everyone-talking-at-once family. I love this aspect the most about my family, but my track record in group conversations was not going all that well, so this would be the ultimate test: sort of like the Conversational Olympics. Perhaps some voice warm-ups and tongue twister exercises would help me prep for the main event?

I had been making steady progress ever since the eye surgery. Challenges abounded, but my recovery was relatively on track. Many of the setbacks were behind us and the trajectory appeared to be going up.

Fate had other plans. A detached retina, to be exact.

Reluctantly, Dr. Kinyoun found the name of a retinal surgeon in Columbus and instructed me to immediately call and get into surgery if my vision degraded further with increased blurriness or "floaters" in my line of sight. He also warned that if I felt my field of vision narrowing, like a telescope collapsing in on itself, I would need immediate surgery and wouldn't have time to fly back.

Paul was not thrilled that I still wanted to go. He'd had enough near-misses with me—this was the last stress he needed. Reassuring him with my doctor referral and list of potential symptoms, I told him we'd be fine. Even if I didn't believe it myself.

Isn't it strange how once you hear a name or a news item mentioned, you start to see it everywhere? Well, once I knew I had a problem, it was like my eye kicked into overdrive.

The next day, I immediately noticed I was having a harder time seeing out of my now good eye. I can't explain it: it wasn't like I saw black. It was just literally like my brain was having trouble processing a picture for what my eye saw. It was like I wasn't quite seeing what I was seeing, as if information was lost between my optic nerve and my brain. I likened this to what it would be like if the *Star Trek* transporter beam had not sent 100 percent of the pixels of the whole person back to the ship.

Simply put, I couldn't see very well.

But we went to the airport anyway. The vision literally got worse from the time I woke up to the time we waited at the gate for our flight. Paul and I played a game of chicken with each other: Should we get onboard? Should we stay? There was no way to know the right answer, because I so desperately wanted to see my family again it was coloring my judgment. I had also made plans to meet up with my best friend and another high school friend I hadn't seen in eighteen years. Given my experience, family and friends meant more to me than ever these days.

We got on board. Funny how a brain injury had not removed one iota of my stubbornness.

On the plane, we decided to immediately call Dr. Kinyoun when we landed and ask him what we should do. My brother Michael happily embraced us at the airport when he picked us up, as he had not seen me since I was in the rehab ward. When we told him the situation, he just shook his head and rolled his eyes. He must have thought we were nuts for even getting on that plane.

Dr. Kinyoun was neither surprised nor ruffled when we called him. I was, by this time, freaking out and pleading, "If we got on a plane tomorrow, would you be able to do the surgery?" I clung to him like a security blanket. After proving himself with the vitrectomy, I was not ready to leave my eyesight to someone who had no real idea of what we'd just been though. Dr. Kinyoun calmly talked me out of it and said that I needed surgery immediately, before the retina completely detached. He said he'd call the surgeon himself and give him a heads up about my case. I think he could sense my fear through the phone line.

Being in the right place at the right time seemed to be a theme throughout this entire ordeal. And, once again, serendipity: the surgeon's office was less than a mile from my brother's house. We made an appointment, zoomed over, and got to explain our whole fun little tale to a new cadre of medical experts: an aneurysm which caused the cerebral hemorrhage which caused the Terson's Syndrome which required a vitrectomy which had caused a detached retina. My health history was starting to sound like a carefully collapsing line of dominos: with one push, the effects seemed to never end.

What I remember most about this office was that the resident who saw me spent almost twenty minutes perfecting a colored-pencil drawing of what he saw in my eye.

I was like, "Really? My eye is about to explode and he's coloring?"

It was excruciating watching him create the sketch and color in the lines like a six-year-old artistic prodigy. Now I was really starting to regret this decision. Later, Dr. Kinyoun was visibly impressed when I shared this information upon returning home: it's actually an old-school way of training eye doctors to understand and map out what is happening in the eye.

This new eye surgeon, a kindly homage to Santa Claus with a white beard and a warm grin, eased my worries with his confidence and clear explanations.

"You've been through quite a lot," he empathized after hearing my tale. He got me into surgery the very next day.

And so the day before Thanksgiving 2008, Paul and I visited another hospital surgery ward and filled out more paperwork. I was introduced to Joe, the anesthesia guy, and was put into "twilight sleep" for the procedure.

He told me, "Now, if you ever feel yourself waking up and want more drugs, just call me and I'll be right there in the room with you."

This was handy, since I do recall coming out a bit during surgery and calling his name. True to his word, I don't remember anything after that.

Waking up in recovery, the searing pain in my eye started as a low hum and then heightened to a feverish crescendo as I came to. It was like the vitrectomy all over again—but not quite as unbearable. Paul was right there at my side as I woke up and, like a good soldier, already knew to have the bowl available for my vomiting. My poor husband normally gags when he sees people throwing up, but he didn't even flinch.

My one good eye was now covered from the surgery so I was back to blurriness and rose petals blocking my vision. Not quite as bad as in the hospital, as it had begun clearing out by now, but still impaired. Frustrated, I felt like I'd just been knocked back three miles. Everything had been going up, up, up. It wasn't perfect, but why the hell did I have to take this stupid step backwards? Was this cycle of hospitals and surgeries ever going to end so I could just get on with my life?

My brother Michael came to see me on a break from his workday as a police sergeant, and he was dressed in full uniform. Nurses stared and whispered as he marched down the hall. "Maybe they'll think there's some famous celebrity staying here," I said.

"Or a felon," quipped my brother, cheering me a bit.

The doctor came to remove the bandage and check things out. My eye was swollen almost completely shut and bruised, as if I'd just gone three rounds with Mike Tyson. But he said it all looked good. I love how doctors can look at a mess like that purple, red and yellow swollen grapefruit on the left side of my face and think it looks good. It makes you wonder what would look not good.

The downside was that this surgery left me with compromised vision In what was currently my only good eye. Whereas the first surgery had not undone the correction from the past Lasik procedure, this one had. I was left a bit near-sighted and blurry and probably in need of a corrective lens.

I got to spend Thanksgiving dinner with my family after all. I didn't want to scare my little nephews and niece, so I donned an eye patch and slowly knocked on the door of my brother's house. The door opened and the four of them streamed out from different rooms to greet us at the front door, but their smiles faded a bit in confusion when they saw the black eye patch.

Thinking fast, I knelt down and bellowed, "Aunt Pirate Maria is here... AAARRRGGGHH, mateys!"

Confusion tuned into huge grins and their chorus of giggles reminded me that, while this was a setback, it was minor.

As we sat down to a feast of juicy honey-colored turkey, sausage stuffing, green beans with garlic and lemon, creamy mashed potatoes—and even our Italian family tradition of antipasto—we said grace. We thanked God for this table, and for being together and for helping me get back to health.

Another thing I love about my family is that while we are sentimental, we stop short of being maudlin. We simply smiled at one another and got down to eating, chatting and laughing about all sorts of crazy things. Which is how we'd approached everything so far: just get on with it, find the humor and keep going.

Later, as we cleared the table, my brother John gave me a big bear hug and I'm sure I felt him shed a tear on my shoulder. But nothing else needed to be said.

Maybe emergency eye surgery was not so bad. I'd already proven I had the strength and acceptance to handle whatever else this crazy situation might throw at me. This was once again a slap upside the head to quit my bitching and to realize that I wasn't even supposed to be here.

I had a helluva lot for which to be thankful. How appropriate for that time of year.

THE SCOTTISH CHRISTMAS TRAVEL ADVENTURE

AFTER THE THANKSGIVING excitement, I started looking forward to our next big trip: Scotland. We had planned to spend Christmas with my in-laws. I was starting to go stir-crazy in Seattle and, while the journey would be challenging, I wanted to see my mother-in-law again and personally thank her for all she did when she came to Seattle. I did not even remember her being here, and that made me sad. In addition, Paul's sister and brother-in-law were flying to Scotland from Connecticut with their kids so that the newest addition, our niece, could be baptized at the village church.

Paul and I were going to spend one romantic night together in London before heading back home. I booked dinner at a great restaurant and a night at a cute little boutique hotel. As you can imagine, there were not many date nights while I was in recovery, even though we did try. It was hard to shift out of caregiver/patient roles and into husband/wife mode on a dime. And I wasn't feeling my most attractive very often anyway, with my shorn head and bony frame.

Ah, Fate. Once again, it had other plans for us. Fate had treated us well in so many respects on this journey. But it also socked us with some ridiculous setbacks.

Winter 2008 was horrible in Seattle. Snow, ice, bitter cold. It's not like this is Chicago, where people know how to handle the ice and snow. Seattle has a lot of hills, just like San Francisco, and ice brings the city to a screeching halt. Buses were late or stopped running. Cars spilled all over the steep hills of our Queen Anne neighborhood. Schools and businesses closed because it was too dangerous for anyone to get around or drive to work.

We were supposed to arrive in London the day before Christmas Eve and hop a regional flight up to Scotland. The Seattle airport was a tangled mess. Ever hopeful, we remained committed. I needed this trip. I needed to get out of the awful weather, forget about the past few months and treat myself to a beautiful Christmas in the Scottish countryside.

We were packed, the dog was in boarding and we were ready to roll. But the morning of our flight, we got the notice that it was delayed three times before it was completely cancelled.

That's when I lost it.

"I want to get out! I just want to get out of here!" Tears streamed down my face as I paced the floor, wringing my hands. Seeing that I was useless, Paul sprang into action and dialed United Airlines.

When all hope seems lost, the compassionate actions of one person can shine light into the darkness. Paul managed to get the kindest customer service rep in a sea of what must have been some harried agents that day. She took pity on us, and rebooked us to London through LA the following day, even though technically we shouldn't have been allowed to do so, due to our fare codes and frequent flier status. She couldn't promise that flight would not get cancelled, but it was a glimmer of hope.

The other challenge was our flight from London to Scotland. Our new flight from LA would make us miss our connection to Inverness, only twenty minutes from Paul's family. The only other flight we were able to get—on Christmas Eve—was to Aberdeen on the other side of the country. An almost three hour drive from where my in-laws live. Good God.

I was exhausted, still fighting my fatigue and unable to handle my frequent roller coaster emotions. I don't know why it was so important for us to go on this trip. I can't explain it. It just felt like my entire recovery depended on it; that if we couldn't make this work, nothing would ever be right again.

But it all worked out. We arrived in London unscathed and made our connecting flight to Scotland. And bless my brother-in-law and father-in-law: they drove almost three hours to pick us up from the Aberdeen airport and turned right around and drove us all back to the house. We arrived near dinnertime.

The one-bathroom house burst with all six of us staying there, plus two kids, two dogs and some persnickety cats. I was never in my life so happy to get to a destination. It was comforting to be surrounded by family, and Paul's mother and I shared a warm embrace when I walked through the door.

Everyone took such good care of me, letting me take much-needed afternoon naps, guiding me carefully over the ice in the church parking lot, making sure I did not exert myself too much. After all, only three months prior, I had a draining tube in my head and a breathing tube down my throat. Plus, I had still not gotten a corrective lens for my left eye yet. But here I was, traveling thousands of miles, despite my frail condition and visual issues. Another reminder of how far I'd come.

The christening was lovely. The weather—not so much. It was foggy and misty and damply cold with plunging temps that are not normal for those parts. But we stayed warm and toasty inside by the fire.

As the final cherry on top on this arduous trip, our carefully planned romantic London night never came to pass. The Inverness airport got fogged in the day we were to leave and all flights were grounded. Paul and I looked at each other, fed up with being at the mercy of the weather and the airlines, and promptly rented a car. We drove ten hours in the bitter cold down to London, arrived at 11 p.m., and took a room at the Heathrow Holiday Inn so we could catch our flight out in the morning. Romantic it was not. Getting home and staying put in Seattle was starting to look very good again.

Nonetheless, the common theme the last few months prevailed. Perhaps Paul and I really could handle any curveballs life wanted to throw at us.

But I think my cabin fever was cured.

IGNORANCE IS BLISS . . . BUT ACCEPTANCE IS DIVINE

"I'LL BOOK A flight today and be there next week."

Upon learning of my vision setback and emergency surgery over Thanksgiving, Carrie had stepped up and offered to come to Seattle. We were in the same boat as we had been when I first came out of the hospital in September—but at least this time I would only need assistance for about a week or so until my eye healed. Relieved at not having to call the in-home babysitters again, I accepted her offer before the words were even out of her mouth.

I was getting good at accepting help. An independent gal, I had always taken care of myself. Living in cities like Chicago, Washington, D.C., and San Francisco on my own, I'd always reveled in my independence. More than that, I hated to inconvenience people. Oddly enough, I was perfectly happy and willing to drop everything if someone needed me, but somehow I struggled to accept that I mattered enough to anyone else for them to do the same.

But after living through this ordeal and getting completely blown away by the outpouring of love and support, I started to practice thankfulness and trust. It was hard at first to accept that I couldn't magically wave a wand and have everything go back to normal. If I was going to ever regain my independence, the irony was that I would have to accept help.

I learned that asking for help in the pursuit of a larger goal is not a sign of weakness. As a new entrepreneur, I was learning this lesson with my business and sought the help of experts and friends who could get me to success faster. The same principle was happening in my personal life, as I relied on others to get back on my feet again.

Since I couldn't drive, I had to rely on friends to pick me up, guide me up and down stairs, and even read small print on menus to me in low-lit restaurants. My friends in book club took turns driving me each month so I would at least get out of the house. I had to rely on therapists to get my strength and stamina back. And I had to rely on Paul for practically everything else.

Having Carrie come out and help for that week was actually a great way for me to be less reliant on Paul. Having someone besides him to lean on was probably the best thing for his stress level as well.

Carrie and I shared a special week. She had not seen me since the hospital and now we could really talk. She gently put drops in my eye twice a day, helped me fix my meals and made sure I didn't fall as I was getting around. Arm in arm, we looked like two chatty old ladies as we walked Eddie down by the canal. And—treat of treats—she even whipped up to-die-for braised short ribs for me, Paul, Guy and Barb one night. Nothing like having a nursemaid who is also a gourmet cook.

I learned, reluctantly, to accept help gracefully (or at least I hope that's how it came off).

But there is another kind of acceptance that was a bigger challenge for me: the acceptance of reality.

After Carrie left and we came home from our Christmas adventure in Scotland, things slowed down. The days turned into an endless stream of waking up, walking the dog and lying on the coach, and they were starting to blur together. In the hospital, the doctors and counselors had gently guided me to set more realistic goals for getting back to work. Their case notes are littered with concerns that I had not grasped the severity of what had happened to me and that this denial might affect my recovery.

You can't heal if you don't know you have a big problem, can you?

"Oh, I'll be able to get back to work in about six or seven weeks," I told one caseworker after another. This, of course, was coming from the same gal who had thought she was still headed for a beach in Spain with a huge scar on her shaved head. Funny. I really believed I was giving myself a nice little vacation by accepting it would be more than six weeks.

My reflections on this…this…what can you call it? Was it stubbornness, ignorance or complete denial? Anyway, with distance, I've been able to laugh at my optimism, shake my head at my naiveté—and, honestly, take some pride in my moxie. But it means more than that.

Why is it that a person can be living life happily and energetically, but once told they have three months to live, deteriorate so rapidly? Is it truly mind over matter?

Scientifically, I don't believe that to always be the case. After all, there have been lots of good people who have succumbed to death or disability and not for lack of faith. Look at Christopher Reeve. He was adamant that he would one day walk again and did everything in his power to try before he passed away. You can't tell me he wasn't stubborn and committed, but the power of his conviction could not overcome his physical constraints.

But there is definitely room to believe that your mental state has as much impact on your health and progress as anything else. How else can you explain so many odds-defying patients who beat breast cancer, overcome physical handicaps, or who are born with congenital diseases who live well past the age their doctors predicted?

Looking back, I think my amazingly rapid recovery had a lot to do with my ignorance of the severity and the odds. I've always been a person who believed that if given a one-in-one-hundred chance of winning something, "Hey, somebody's gotta be that 'one,' right? Why not me?" Odds are there for a reason. Some people beat them, some don't.

Could this Pollyanna attitude also explain my love for playing craps in Vegas?

I didn't know how serious my health situation was. In the hospital, I couldn't check the internet. I couldn't read the reports. Carrie had dived into an internet full of cranial research but instead of getting lost in the numbers, she actually used that knowledge to be a strong patient advocate for me and to ask intelligent questions about my continuity of care.

"I do remember early on having various conversations about whether or not people wanted to see statistics," Carrie said. "The odds were, frankly, pretty dire and we all knew that on some level. I remember deciding to look at the stats and having that first howling grief, but I don't think I ever doubted it would somehow be fine. Just because it had to be, I guess, and not because it made any logical sense that it would be."

That's about the best way I can explain my frame of mind. It was never a question of *if* but always a question of *when*, as far as I was concerned. And in that single-minded focus, there was no time or room for maudlin "Why me?" questions either.

We humans ask ourselves that question a lot, don't we? *Why did this tragic event happen to me? Why do I have to suffer fools? Why does it always rain when I've forgotten my umbrella?*

But I've never quite been able to get on board with this concept. While I'm blissfully optimistic and positive, I am also a realist. Okay, my current tale is not a good example of this realism, but I'm usually the person focused on this question instead: "Why *not* me?"

What makes me so special that it should be someone else suffering instead of me? Asking "Why me?" seems an incredibly selfish and fruitless waste of time.

The conversation changes, however, when you upend the question and ask, "Why not me?" You go from victim to leader; from "I could never..." to "Damn straight, I will!" You start focusing on solutions and not whining about problems.

I was determined not to whine. Not admitting weakness in those early days of recovery meant I was going to be fine and I'd handle it all. And that soon I'd be back on the train of my crazy life again.

But none of that was going to happen with me vegging on the couch, watching game shows and bad daytime TV.

Having initially targeted January as my get-back-to-work month, I quickly realized it was not going to happen. I couldn't even get down to my office to log on to email. For about a week, I tried. I really did. I wrote down my goal: just go downstairs, log on and respond to emails for about ten minutes. That's it. No problem. I should have been able to do that in my sleep.

Each day started with that intent. I'd shower. I'd dress. I'd walk Eddie. I'd even read the paper. Yet I couldn't bring myself to head downstairs to my office. Or I got distracted by reading the paper for too long. Or I'd find some other reason to not do what I'd planned to do that day. I just couldn't initiate action and get my motor running. Paul would get home around 5 p.m. and find me curled up with a blanket and Eddie, almost in tears, not understanding what the hell was wrong with me. This was going nowhere. I needed help...and fast.

I was slated to start outpatient rehab therapy groups in early 2009. For eight weeks, the plan was to meet on Tuesdays with a group devoted to cognitive strategies: memory, attention, focus, comprehension. On Thursdays, a smaller group discussed psychotherapy issues: depression, irritability, mood swings and anxiety. I was actually excited to attend these groups and get to work on fixing myself. But I needed to conquer the demons in my own house one on one with someone before dealing with other patients in similar dire straits.

Once again, the lesson of learning to ask for help showed up in my life. We called Rehab Without Walls again and asked if they could send a speech therapist back for a few sessions to help me overcome my initiation issues and put me on an achievable schedule. Our insurance approved the sessions and we were set.

My therapist Jane and I hit it off immediately, and I could tell this was going to be an important step in my recovery. She listened to my bewildered accounts of what was happening to me and explained that it was important to get me onto a set schedule.

Brain injury patients, especially those with frontal lobe injuries, need a foundation to which to cling, she explained. A healthy brain can clear away all the stimuli and focus on what is important. My damaged brain was reading every single input as the same priority—and it was paralyzing me into inaction as a result. A schedule would help me focus and more easily silence all the voices demanding my attention at the same time.

We met in my office, not upstairs, to get me used to being next to my computer and in my chair. She helped me craft a weekly schedule that included my morning routine and some measurable goals, such as time spent on email or the number of coffee dates I would attend in a given week.

Sounds simple, right?

But it was like the sun burst into my cloudy day. I don't know if it was her education and experience with what was happening to me, or her reassurance that what I was going through was normal given my brain injuries, but it helped me get past trying to make sense of it all and just adapt.

Acceptance. That lesson was key to getting me through the rest of my recovery.

Before this, I had seen everything as so black and white. "If I say I'm brain injured, I won't ever get back to my life, so I'll minimize the injury as much as possible and just push through."

I had thought admitting to change meant I was broken.

What I learned from Jane was that there was going to be a New Me. Not better or worse, but new. I could fight it all I wanted, but the sooner I accepted this new reality, the sooner I could adapt and deal with it.

Acceptance doesn't mean giving up. It's seeing the reality in front of you and making the best out of the situation. This actually meshed well with my "Why *not* me?" philosophy, but I had lost sight of it. To me, getting well had meant getting back to the old baseline again. Not true.

It was now a new playing field. Getting healthy meant that I needed to honestly assess the obstacles and then see how far I could knock them over or how I could zip around them instead.

Jane let some light into that darkness so I could realize it was not about the Old Me. It was about the here and now and making the New Me work.

Working with her rebooted my system and my approach to recovery. This turning point of asking for help completely rewired my thinking.

Specifically, Jane knew I was frustrated with my slow reactions to conversation and vocabulary. In pursuit of this, she turned me on to a fantastic mind-games website called Lumosity (www.lumosity.com), which is full of games to help keep a person's brain sharp as it gets older.

Playing off of my love for trivia and board games, this was the perfect way to flex my cognitive muscles. I did the Word Bubble game, in which the computer showed me a letter and I had so much time to come up with as many words that began with that letter as I could. I also practiced a spatial relationship game: a bird briefly flashed somewhere on the screen and I had to pay close attention and click the mouse over the place where I'd just seen it appear.

The various games kept me engaged and at my desk, and in front of my computer for a set amount of time every day. Clever.

Most importantly, the games brought tiny little victories that my psyche desperately needed. I thrive on momentum. A body in motion stays in motion, and all of that.

Finally, at the end of each day, I felt like I had accomplished something. Not surprisingly, this led me to want to do more and more. It got me over the "initiation hump."

"I got the most words I've ever gotten at Word Bubbles today!" I often cried with glee when Paul came home from work.

He was happy to see my smile again.

GETTING MY GROUP THERAPY ON

Taking the bus with my vision impairments was like stepping into an abyss every time and hoping things turned out all right. They always did—but not without completely stressing me out.

Since I couldn't drive, the bus system became my new best friend. With the vision problems I had at the time, my occupational therapist helped me navigate which bus would take me to the hospital for follow-up appointments. She walked me the two blocks from my house to the closest bus stop and, using directions she'd printed out in advance, ensured I could recognize where I needed to disembark. Even though it was early 2009, my one-eyed vision was still blurry due to the retinal surgery a few months prior. I learned to make out the trees and the layout of the bus stop where I needed to exit the bus. To avoid any transfers, we disembarked in what seemed like a grove of trees at the University of Washington campus' bus transfer depot, walked across an overpass to the Health Sciences Building near the Medical Center, and then made our way through a labyrinth of hallways to the adjacent hospital itself. Add in a few elevator bank switches and it could not have been more complicated for me.

Slowly, carefully, after taking a wrong turn and ending up in a corridor of deserted lockers, I found my way by myself to my first cognitive group therapy session. Finally finding the right meeting room, I grabbed the closest seat I could find.

I didn't talk to anyone; I wasn't the normal, smiley Maria I usually am when in new groups. I clung to my chair so tightly, my knuckles turned white. Since everyone was a bit blurry, I focused on my pad of paper in front of me instead.

We were to meet for eight weeks with a clinical rehab psychologist and a speech therapist. After they welcomed us, we went around the room and introduced ourselves. But instead of the normal fun-fact ice breaker that's typical in new groups, our task was to tell the group what caused our brain injury and when it had happened.

As we made our way through fifteen attendees, I was struck by the diversity of circumstances. Brain tumor. Stroke. Aneurysm. Hit by a car. Motorcycle crash.

Some people had experienced their injuries years ago. Some, like me, were still growing back our hair. Some had traveled from other cities just to attend UW's nationally-recognized rehab center. And, sadly, some came with walkers and others had trouble forming words or had to repeat themselves because their speech was not easily understood.

What on earth am I doing here? I thought to myself.

I had been in denial about the severity of my trauma, as well as any long lasting effects, for so long that I didn't realize how lucky I'd been. But for the grace of God, I could have been any one of these people.

Some had lost friends who didn't understand why they were the way they were now. Others couldn't drive anymore due to the anti-seizure medication they were now on. One man was a successful research doctor who might never be able to practice medicine again due to his brain damage.

Sobered by their stories and their circumstances, I quickly wrapped myself further inward to protect myself, selfishly not wanting to let any of it rub off on me.

Along with feeling selfish, I felt guilty. I was absolutely hunky-dory when compared to many of these brave folks. But as they talked about the issues they were having since their injuries, I perked up as I heard descriptions of all-too-familiar symptoms:

I can't get up off the couch. I used to get so much done in a day, but I've lost my get up and go. My wife thinks that I've become lazy and irresponsible.

I was in sales and used to be excellent at names. Now I can meet someone five times and still not recall their name.

I'm afraid to be alone sometimes. I get so anxious about being by myself, but then I also get anxious when I leave the house and there's too much going on around me.

I struggle to find the right words when I'm talking. I know what I want to say, but I can't find the right way to say it.

I can't focus on a dinner conversation when I'm at a restaurant. My mind wanders or I can't help but overhear all the other conversations going on around me. It's frustrating!

Whoa. Seriously? Get out of my head!

These were exactly the things I was struggling with on a daily basis.

Our group leaders nodded empathetically and told us what we all needed to hear. "These are all common and normal effects of brain injury that we see over and over again."

Hallelujah.

"In this Tuesday group, we're going to help you improve speaking, thinking and comprehension skills in everyday interactions. And for most of you, the Thursday group sessions will explore some of the emotional and psychological aspects of what you're dealing with, so it will be a nice complement. But our group will focus on understanding your cognitive strengths and weaknesses so you can learn strategies to adapt to them and function without frustration."

Bring it, I thought. Eight weeks of this, and I'll be back to full-time work in no time.

Um. Yeah. Right.

The best part of our group session was the ground rules. Our leaders explained that many brain injury patients tend to lack self-regulation when it comes to behavior. It's like your filter is damaged: you may ramble on (hyperverbality), wander aimlessly off point (tangentiality) or say something blunt or socially inappropriate. This last one was jokingly referred to as "losing your social graces."

"One of our rules is that if you go off-topic or seem to be dwelling on points that are taking us away from the main focus, we will interrupt you and we'll gently steer you back on track. Please don't take this personally, because we do this for your benefit and the benefit of the group."

Um, can we make this a rule at every single work meeting ever conducted in the history of Corporate America? This was awesome! You actually had an excuse for making somebody stop rambling and get back to the task at hand.

Over the next eight weeks, we learned about the most common cognitive effects that patients mention after brain injury. Learning about these effects was like having the fog and rain lift and the sun stream through the window. It was an immediate relief and validation for what I'd been going through and feeling. Aliens had not invaded my body after all. I was *supposed* to be tired, cranky and lazy.

Hitches in My Brain's "Cognitive Giddy'up"

According to University of Washington rehabilitation group materials[18], some of the most popular cognitive effects patients mention after brain injury—and many of which I experienced firsthand due to my frontal lobe injury—include the following:

- *Reduced attention and concentration*
- *Heightened distractibility*
- *Memory problems and reduced new learning capacity*
- *Slowness in thinking and performance*
- *Problems in flexibility of thinking*
- *Difficulties with planning, organizing and initiation*
- *Reduced abstract reasoning capacity*
- *Impaired complex information processing skills*
- *Problems in judgment*

- *Visual spatial and visual perception impairments (for example, directions, path-finding, mechanical skills, location of objects in space)*
- *Low fatigue threshold*
- *Communication disturbances, including verbal expansiveness and tangentiality*
- *Basic intellectual deficits as measured by IQ*
- *Confusion and perplexity*

The item "problems in flexibility of thinking" especially resonated with me. This explained my severely emotional reaction to the unexpected and constant changes in our Christmas travel plans. Or why I reacted so badly when I thought we were running one set of errands and Paul changed the plan on me at the last minute. Or why a change in meeting location would throw me into a tizzy of doubt and fear. I'd never been so set in my ways before, but it was almost as if my new dependence of keeping a schedule (which had helped in the early days) tilted me so far over onto the planning side that any change could seriously upset my whole day.

Partly, this was my type A personality rearing its ugly head, but it had never been that bad before. I now knew why I was feeling this way. It was such a huge relief to know it was real and explainable.

Now all I had to do was learn to adapt.

We learned many strategies over the next eight weeks. That's a big word in therapy: *strategies*. Paul and I used to say in a mocking tone to each other, "What's my *strategy* going to be for handling this barbecue/party/plane trip?"

"I'm a delicate flower now. You must do everything I say or my brain might explode again," I said, regally thrusting my chin up in the air.

"How long are you going to play that brain-injury card?" Paul laughed back.

"As long as I can."

Good old humor. The strategy that works every time.

In our Tuesday group meetings, we learned how to take good notes when someone is speaking. We learned how to manage our time and organize our calendar each day by blocking out time for therapy, naps, personal errands and breaks along with our work. We learned how to practice focusing on the conversation in front of us and asking clarifying questions to stay engaged. We learned about leaving notepads within reach to jot down reminders and useful information so we wouldn't forget. We learned how to reduce distractions in our work and home lives by setting timers, turning off email notifications, or turning down the radio. We learned about checklists and alarms and taking breaks and asking for clarification.

Basically, it was a crash course in communications, effective listening, time management and project management all rolled into one.

I felt extremely lucky to be a college-educated, white-collar professional. Many of these tips and tricks were things I had already learned in workshops, professional training, or from reading Stephen Covey. I could tell some of these concepts were brand spanking new to many of my fellow group members, though, and it was a lot for them to digest. Just as I had during the neuropsych test, I ached for those in less fortunate circumstances than mine. How do they handle it?

The Thursday sessions dealt with more emotional and psychological issues—in other words, very personal and tough ones. We met in a small room with only five fellow group members, a rehab counselor and a clinical neuropsychologist. These folks were in my cognitive rehab group as well.

While the mood in the cognitive groups was practical and congenial, entering this room was like walking into a wake. Speaking in hushed tones, the somber mood made the hair on the back of my neck stand on end.

"We want to help you understand the emotional changes brought on by your brain injury and to help you with coping strategies," the leaders said.

I felt like some deep, dark, ancient secret was about to be revealed, so I might better understand where my fear, anxiety, anger and frustration were coming from.

Like with the cognitive group, I was looking for solutions. There had to be a way to "fix" me, I thought.

These sessions focused on our moods and emotions, and constructive ways to handle fear, anger and other negative emotions. Where the cognitive group was all about practical daily life, this group focused more on the inside.

How were our brains dealing with what had happened to them?

The Jekyll and Hyde Effects of Brain Injury

Brain injury doesn't just affect cognition. That's where the psychotherapy group came in. We dealt with organically-based personality changes, which are a direct result of the brain injury, and emotional reactions, which are psychological responses to the injury, not a direct result of the brain damage. I was shocked to learn from my University of Washington Medical Center reference materials that brain injury can cause these effects in our personality and mood.[19]

Common, organically-based personality changes that result directly from brain injury can include:

- *Impulsivity*
- *Unrealistic self-appraisal*
- *Disinhibition (related to that filter loss I mentioned earlier)*
- *More easily frustrated*
- *Suspiciousness or paranoia*
- *Misperceive other people's intentions or actions*
- *Reduced or altered sense of humor*
- *Reduced capacity for empathy*
- *Rage reactions*
- *Rapid and dramatic mood swings*
- *Inappropriate or uncontrolled laughing or crying*
- *Childlike reactions or behavior*
- *Difficulty starting or stopping a particular behavior*

As a result of these direct challenges, common emotional reactions to the brain injury itself can include:

- *Reduced self-esteem*
- *Withdrawal*
- *Sadness*
- *Anger, irritability*
- *Grief*
- *Anxiety*
- *Depression*
- *Humiliation, embarassment*
- *Increased sense of dependence on others*
- *Fear of being alone*
- *Resistance, defensiveness*
- *Hopelessness*
- *Helplessness*
- *Preoccupation with the past*
- *Unrealistic expections of family and friends*

This Thursday group dealt with the stuff no one can see from your physical state. Instead, others might think you've become childish or cold or an asshole. They might not relate it to the brain injury at all.

I will never forget one of the men in my group. I'll call him Lawson. He was a sweet guy who'd had a brain injury a while back and was desperate to get help. His changed behavior had led to major misunderstandings and a pending divorce with his wife. At one session, he exclaimed, "I'm going to show her this binder so she'll finally understand! She just thinks I'm being lazy and moody, but I keep telling her I don't understand why I'm acting this way."

Heartbreaking. Once again, I threw a silent "thank you" heavenward for my understanding and intelligent husband.

But who among us really knows the effects of brain injury until we're forced to? Paul and I got to learn more about the brain than we ever cared to know, and now I get why parents are up in arms about sports and head injuries. You just never know what that bump, collision or crash is going to impact down the road. I once heard a medical story on TV about a very angry man who started drinking a lot and shouted at his family all the time. He was a nightmare to live with and his kids—now adults—noted that they could remember a time when he didn't act this way. This personality change had completely damaged his relationship with his children. Years later, he finally went for a head scan and they found an old brain injury from when he had fallen off a ladder. Unfortunately, it was one of those "I'm fine, I'll shake it off" moments that led to catastrophic results when it didn't have to.

Accepting feedback and addressing these challenges is vital to rehabilitation. You have to hear the feedback in order to do anything about it. One of the harder tasks in the psychotherapy group was that Paul had to read the information in our binder and write down which changes and reactions he felt I was exhibiting—and not only that, but provide examples.

He didn't want to do this at first. He was so afraid of upsetting me. But in the end, he knew he had to help me get better and that started with being honest.

While we had talked about much of this, seeing it in Paul's handwriting was sobering:

More easily frustrated. For example, she always thinks other drivers are getting in our way on purpose, and she yells that they are bad drivers (more so than she used to). She also can't stand when insignificant plans change, like when we run errands in a different order or make something for dinner other than what we'd planned.

Unrealistic self-appraisal. For example, she underestimates her abilities or lacks confidence. She is much more hesitant than she was before, and she doesn't trust herself.

Overreaction. Lots of small issues seem to blow up.

Inconsistent behavior. Her assessment of a situation seems to change rapidly from anger to confusion to acceptance and back again.

Lack of initiative. She often shows very little initiative to do things if she's not being pushed, which is not like her.

As for emotional issues, he cited my fear of being alone, and my irritability, sadness, hopelessness and depression.

What was to be done? How could I *fix* this?

Well, part of our time in this group was spent talking about grief and loss after a brain injury. We reviewed the common stages of grief as identified by Elizabeth Kubler-Ross. Seeing the examples of how each stage manifests as a script in your head was like a lightning bolt for me. While I was not affected so much by the "rage or anger" stage, I totally recognized myself in the denial, bargaining and depression stages:

Denial. You are not ready to accept that life may be different, and so you allow yourself to think that you will be back to your old self.

Bargaining. "If I give myself another month, I know I will be able to do all the things I used to. I just need more time."

Depression. "I am extremely sad about my situation."

I saw depression in my quieter moments, when I could not get off the couch. My energy was drained and I wanted to hide away from the world.

In my frustration over not being able to find the right word or to remember an important message or to tackle my to-do list, I often wondered, "Who am I? Who is this strange person in my body who can't do the things she used to be so good at? *Who am I supposed to be now?*"

This is when the light of acceptance dawned on me once more. *Remember, Maria, you are learning about all of this. You now know what is happening inside your head. You can now fix the problem.*

But there was not going to be any "fixing." It was about ceasing the childish kicking and screaming and accepting that things were different.

Between the bleeding that sliced through my brain cells like a knife, and the vasospasms that caused a loss of blood flow and oxygen for a bit, some tissue in my brain had died. It was never coming back.

So what did I have to work with now?

We focused a lot on identifying and dealing with negative emotions. We wrote about past successes and the personality traits that had contributed to them, so we could remind ourselves of what we still had. We learned a technique to identify and change unhealthy thoughts. When we found ourselves facing a negative situation, we learned to calm ourselves down, examine the emotions and the "evidence," come up with alternate thoughts or scenarios, and then assess our new emotional outcome.

I love the following example, since this is exactly what I was thinking and feeling:

What is the situation? I always took pride in working hard and being productive. Since my brain injury, I find I am tired almost all of the time and everything takes so much longer to do.

Rate my emotions on a scale of 1 to 10: overwhelmed (9), angry (9), depressed (8).

What are the unhealthy thoughts I have? "I can't possibly do more. It takes all I have just to go to all my therapy and doctor appointments. I should be able to do more. Why can't I manage such simple things? I'm useless."

Reframe into an adaptive thought. "I can't expect more of myself right now. My priority and focus is to get better to whatever degree is possible. I am working as hard as I can. I see progress but it may take longer than I expected. My spouse is overwhelmed, too. I will explain to him that I can't do all the things he requested. Maybe we can agree on what is the most important thing for me to help with."

Rate my new emotional outcomes, or a scale of 1 to 10: overwhelmed (7), angry (5), depressed (5).

This was acceptance in action. It was taking the situation for what it was, reframing it, and then moving forward. I may not get back to my old state of normal, but I sure as hell can adapt around the obstacles.

Mostly, rehab gave me relief. Relief that I was "normal" in this abnormal situation.

Relief that what I was going through was common.

And relief that I would find a way to deal with it, to manage it and to move on.

FLYING SOLO

"So, DO YOU think I can get Lasik surgery on my eye yet?" I asked Dr. Kinyoun eagerly at one of my regular vision check-ups in early February.

Having worn contact lenses since I was thirteen, I had invested in the corrective eye surgery known as Lasik four years earlier and it changed my life. No more contact cases! No more disinfecting solution! No more trying to figure out what to do when camping or swimming.

The November retinal reattachment surgery had undone some of the Lasik correction in my left eye. As a result, my one good eye was actually quite blurry after that surgery, which obviously made getting around harder than it had to be. I was eager to get it corrected again as soon as possible.

He did his usual poking, prodding and testing, and then announced, "Well, look at that. You have a cataract."

Screech. That damn record skipped again.

"So what does that mean?"

"As I mentioned when your retina detached, our eyes don't generally like when we muck around in there," he said. "Your eye has had a lot of distress in these last few months, so between the damage and the two surgeries, it seems to have caused a cataract."

"Does that mean I can't get Lasik now?"

"It means you should probably see if you need cataract surgery first or not," he said. "Cataract surgery on the lens could correct the vision, which means you wouldn't need Lasik. I'm going to send you to my colleague at the Refractive Surgery Center for verification. She'll be able to tell you more about if and when you need to operate on this."

"Well, I need to do something about my vision, so should I just go ahead and get a contact lens for this eye to correct things until I see what's up?"

"Sure," said Dr. Kinyoun. "I'll refer you to another colleague who can fit you for a contact in that eye to correct your vision in the interim. But just know that, with a cataract, your vision will change and get progressively worse, so you may need additional prescriptions as your eye worsens."

Lovely.

My glorious four-plus years of corrective-lens-free living had come to an end. Ah well. I'd had a brain aneurysm. Seriously, the consequences could be worse.

Sure enough, the specialist made her diagnosis. I did indeed have a cataract, but it was not yet bad enough to do surgery on. It was pointless to pay for Lasik when we had no idea when I'd need cataract surgery, so it would simply be an issue of monitoring. Just like my brain.

I had held off for so long in the hopes of just getting permanent corrective surgery. With that option off the table for a while, I relented and went to the third doctor to get fitted for a contact lens. When he placed that miraculous little plastic disk in my left eye, I rapidly blinked it into place and stared at the eye chart.

Sweet Jesus, *I could see it!* Clearly. In detail. The outlines of the letters. The black figures starkly outlined against the white background, without blurring together.

I looked around in the small exam room. I could crisply see the rich detail of the books, instruments and papers lining the shelf. Why had I waited so long?

At that moment, I didn't care less about lens cases or contact solution. A light turned on and my blurry world sharpened into focus. I was like one of those students who is failing because she can't read the blackboard and suddenly starts realizing everything she was missing and gets straight As.

So while the cataract was in itself a setback—and meant more eye surgeries in my future—finally moving forward and getting the contact lens I so desperately needed was a breakthrough. I could still only predominantly see out of one eye. But now that eye was fit, clear and ready for action.

Denial sucks. Only when I finally gave myself permission to accept my condition and stop waiting to return to my old self was I able to get to the next level. Getting my sight corrected did wonders for removing the fear and dread when I went out on my own.

I was ready for my next challenge: traveling without Paul.

Becky had her baby in January 2009. A gorgeous little girl. She had done so much for me and Paul, I really wanted to see her. That February, I chose to go to New York City and visit her for a long weekend.

Me. On a plane. By myself. I was petrified. But I knew I had to take this important step. As a former road warrior, I used to fly all over the place for work. Now I couldn't seem to leave the house without a panic attack. I had to visit Becky to prove to myself that I could. And I had to try and do it without Paul. He needed a break. And I needed to find my independence again.

Paul was just as nervous as I was. This was the first time I'd be out of his sight since the injury. Once you find your spouse on the floor unconscious, it's hard not to picture your loved one having another relapse when you're not around. I was still fighting fatigue but I knew I could do this.

Anxious and fearful, I boarded the plane and made my way to New York. At JFK, the chaos was deafening. Voices shouted in various languages, and random bells and announcements fought for air space over the intercom. People streamed up and down the concourse, jostling, running, changing directions.

I hugged the wall, with my eyes focused on my feet in front of me. This trick of focusing on one stage of the journey at a time seemed to be working.

Deplane. Find baggage claim. Get bag.

My aunt was picking me up and I was going to spend a night with her before heading to Becky's in Manhattan. I made my way outside and, with shaking hands, called my aunt to find out where she was.

Balanced on the platform, I peered with my one good eye into the throng of cars, taxis and buses. I didn't even know what her car looked like! Breathing slowly in and out, I found a safe spot to wait and scan the oncoming cars. It felt like hours. Would I be able to see her face through the windshield? What if she couldn't pull over to the curb in time?

Using my behavioral strategies from rehab, I reframed the negative thoughts:

If I don't see her, she'll see me or she'll call.
If she can't pull over right away, she'll circle around and come back again.
She won't leave the airport without me!

I realize most people can reframe negative thought patterns unconsciously by viewing them through the lens of reality. I mean, of course she wasn't going to just leave the airport without me. That's silly. It was just that I had to consciously talk myself through the rational thought process or risk a panic attack. I had to assist my internal filter with silencing the rest of the noise so I could focus on one thing at a time.

Nothing dramatic happened, of course. She found me, I had a great weekend and it was a joy to be able to laugh and talk with Becky—and remember it this time. I was still floored that she had been at my bedside and I never knew it. To boot, my friend Elizabeth was also in town so I got to thank both of them with lots of hugs and smiles for everything they did for me.

I felt like a refreshed person after that trip. Socially, I still had some things to work through, but I had done it. I'd regained my independence and confidence to some degree. I'd tackled NYC, for goodness sake!

That trip gave me the confidence boost I needed to try the next major hurdle: getting back to work.

THE NEW ME GOES BACK TO WORK

In February 2009, while I started group rehab session and began learning strategies for my new deficits, I also dipped my toe back into the work waters.

While therapists suggested I take on a less risky pro-bono volunteer project to gauge my abilities, I took on an exciting project for a friend that we thought would only be about ten, maybe twenty hours per week. Contrary to all criteria the therapists had advised, it was completely unstructured, chaotic and without clear boundaries or rules.

So the ten to twenty hours ended up taking the "New Me" much, much longer than anticipated. I had to manage a huge sales effort and spreadsheet of names, develop templates and tools that didn't exist, keep track of hundreds of emails, calls, and varying stages of paperwork and payment for over 500 businesses. It was mayhem. It would normally be mayhem in a good way for me, but most days, I cried because I was completely overwhelmed. What should I tackle next? Did that person send back her form to me? Did I respond to her question about payment terms? Did I or didn't I send that email I meant to send to those ten businesses?

Normally someone who thrives on adrenaline and this type of buzz, I couldn't think on my feet as fast as I used to, couldn't react quickly enough to the new inputs coming at me every day. Some days I'd literally be paralyzed by it all and would just sit at my desk, staring at the computer and bawling my eyes out.

Stimuli overload seemed to be my biggest problem. The best way to explain this is that the Old Me used to have a suave and efficient bouncer standing at the door to the club that was my brain. He let in only VIPs from among all those clamoring for attention behind the velvet rope. It didn't matter how pushy or loud the line became: the bouncer would only let in a few people at a time and, once inside, the vibe was dynamic yet orderly. Guests could settle into their couches, order their cocktails and breathe a sigh of relief not to be stuck in the cacophony outside.

The bouncer at the door of New Me's brain was pretty green. He fumbled for his clipboard, couldn't answer questions, and got knocked around. People pushed past him or even snuck right by. The result was that the club was overrun by people clamoring this way and that, and security staff didn't know who to chase first. The lights, the crowd, the throbbing beat of the music—it was pandemonium, and I just wanted to find a corner and hide.

My brain could no longer filter extra information: it took it all in with equal weight. At once. Where I used to be able to pay attention to a conference call while checking my email, jotting notes and drinking tea, now I was a one-trick pony. Any outside stimulation distracted my attention and focus, which meant tasks that used to be a cakewalk for me, like crafting a thoughtful sales letter or creating a project plan, ended up taking much longer than they ever did before.

The flip side of this issue was that, once I was finally able to focus, I often couldn't turn it off. Some days I went from nine in the morning to six at night without stopping for lunch. Paul often had to force me to shut down the computer and drag me upstairs from my desk to come eat dinner in the evenings.

It scared the hell out of me.

This was the first time I confronted how my brain injury impacted my professional sense of self. I had always been a top performer and if I couldn't handle this project, I wasn't sure what my future consulting career would hold for me. I might be like one of those folks in my rehab group who couldn't go back to the career they'd had. Had I lost my entrepreneurial and strategic business mojo? Would I end up having to work in a predictable, highly-scoped job with lots of standardized processes, like a barista or a data entry clerk? I had no idea.

I started putting the strategies I was learning in my therapy groups to work on this project. Start from the beginning, I told myself. Forget everything else and, just like with my recovery, break it down into steps. Now, order those steps....

Pretty soon, I had the bones of a plan in front of me. If I could not be handed a project plan on a silver platter, than I was going to create one myself that would work for the New Me.

I turned my email notifications off while I was on the phone. I tried clearing my desk except for tasks on which I was immediately working, but because of my memory issues, I had to keep things in front of me so they would not be forgotten. I tested various folders and organizational systems to stay efficient. Having been a neat person my whole life, this had never been a problem before but I couldn't deal with this clutter around me (again, too much stimuli). So I learned to organize in new ways—and keep items out of my sight but still accessible when working or writing.

Being forced to focus and slow down is not a bad thing at all. Focusing my time and energy on one task at a time was really a blessing, especially in our age of rapid response and 24/7 media stimulation. They say our brains are being re-wired—in a bad way—with all the multitasking that people are forced to do these days, so maybe I was ahead of the curve on this one. My focus was now on quality over quantity. Where I once might have blazed through a myriad of work and communications without thinking, I was now savoring each task that I completed.

Part of this reframing also involved being okay with saying no. I'm a classic over-committer. But I couldn't do that anymore. I had to make choices. I needed to make a firm decision about the clients I accepted and which ones would be time or energy sucks for me. It's hard as a business owner to say no to new clients or partners, but I had to in order to survive.

If I spent my entire time saying yes to the *wrong* things, I wouldn't be able to spend time saying yes to the *right* things. *Quality over quantity* became my new mantra.

I also reframed the mental conversations that chipped away at my self-esteem during this crucial comeback period. Using the techniques I'd learned, I took out my worksheets and wrote the current negative situation and how to deal with it. Instantly, my thinking cleared, my pulse slowed down and I could forge ahead.

I successfully completed this project. Paul forced me to celebrate all of my tiny victories along the way with a massage or by taking a break and getting a latte.

"Look at what you've done, Maria!" he said. "You made all of these sales, you put all of these processes in place for the client. You made all of these people happy. *And you had a brain aneurysm only seven months ago!*"

Nothing can silence the doubt in your head faster than an outside party pointing out how far you've come. When we got my first check for this new project, we did a happy dance and went out for dinner. Victories, however tiny, need to be savored.

Having my own business turned out to be a godsend. I could ramp up at my own pace and the only person I had to answer to was myself. With my newfound acceptance to focus, I could also decide how many clients I could handle at one time.

Because of this reduced workload, I was able to tackle a project I'd wanted for a while. I began writing a short e-book outlining how a business owner could build a strong brand and marketing strategy. This was the perfect project for me, as I was revisiting old material—sharpening my saw, if you will. I could write when I felt like it or until I got tired. And it was a nice mental boost to show myself that I still knew my craft well and had what it took.

Had I been going down the track I'd been on before the injury, with my non-stop schedule, constant pressure and taking on too much, I'm not sure I ever would have made time to create this e-book. Beaming with pride, I put the finishing touches on the e-book's format and uploaded it to my website for sale that April.

I guess this project was my way of testing my marketing knowledge and assuring myself that I could still add value. Business owners responded positively to it, and experts I had never met connected with me on social media to tell me how much they loved it. This external validation was a huge salve to my wounded psyche.

If I wasn't in recovery, would I ever have sat down to write it? I'm not sure. But as with so much in this chapter of my life, I was exactly where I was meant to be at exactly the right time. Things really do happen for a reason.

I'm not advising that you wait for a near-fatal brain injury to follow your dreams. But I have to acknowledge that some things in my life were propelled into action as a result. Life is like that: both good and bad events shove us along. As it turned out, this e-book played a crucial role in accomplishing a larger dream of mine later that year.

I knew I still needed my psychotherapy group to deal with my emotional effects. But I tried to opt out of the last two weeks of cognitive group rehab. While I'd learned so much, I felt like many of the skills they were teaching us were things I already knew and just needed to put into practice. My time would be better spent focusing on this work project and reconnecting with my business network, I thought.

The group leaders, however, must have seen my kind of denial before. They felt I'd benefit from finishing out the group class both for myself and for the others in the class. "People look up to you, Maria. You are not only helping yourself, but you help give them something to strive for, too. You're a great role model for them."

What? Huh? I was helping *them?* Didn't they know *they* inspired *me?* Some of those folks were so much worse off than I was, and yet there they were. Fighting, learning, trying.

This was the first inkling that my experience and story might help other people. While I was stubbornly trying to make my way back up into the saddle of my life, I never stopped to think that some people can't and don't think that way.

One friend even told me, "If this had happened to me, I think I might have used the brain injury as an excuse to hide away and not attempt anything. But you just fought to get right back into the game again."

When you get yanked out of your life—by crisis, death, illness or catastrophe—it's hard enough to get back on track. But when part of what yanked you out actually impacts your initiation, focus and mood, it's like a double whammy.

I think the secret is part stubbornness, part denial and part pure gumption. And having a support system—and amazing resources—to kick your butt quite a bit along the way.

My point is, *fight.* Fight as hard as you can against the inertia, the self-pity, the doubt and the fear.

I'm not suggesting you fight reality like I did at first—it's about *accepting* reality and working with it. But play to your strengths. Don't listen to anyone who tries to define you by your deficits. Learn how to work around them.

I had to learn what the hell was going on with my brain and my personality before I could deal with it. I had to name it, find the root cause, and educate myself. Once I accepted the reality of what had changed, even if no one could see it except for me, I was in a much better position to push past it and evolve.

It was pointless to cry over what I used to be able to do, or question why things were so hard now. I could whine and complain about it or I could adapt. The past was in the past. I was lucky and still had so many gifts yet to give, and I had to figure out how to offer them to the world in a whole new way.

Life is going to throw some nasty crap at you. When it does, you can curl up in a corner and hide, or you can accept the new reality and adapt your life accordingly, even if that means trying every possible strategy on God's green earth.

FACING THE FEAR

ONCE I LEARNED that my brain injury effects were somewhat common and expected, you would think my confidence would blossom. Fear, however, was a huge ugly monster that visited me daily. This was a houseguest I was not used to having around.

Given my rocky transition from patient to self-reliant individual, given the trauma I went through, and given some of the personality and cognitive changes, I didn't know which way was up. Who was I in this new reality and how would I define myself? I was scared about who I was and what I was capable of doing as I tested the boundaries each day.

As a very independent gal, this new dependence on people was like visiting a foreign country and not knowing the language. Every moment, you're on high alert and using tons of brain power and energy to get by.

It's not only scary, it's exhausting.

Paul had been ever-present while I was recovering and had made most of the decisions. While I was eager to restore the balance in our roles and relationship, I was also anxious and panicky. You may want the training wheels taken off the bike, but it doesn't mean you're any less scared when it happens.

I wasn't the only one who was scared. Paul had his own fears, mostly of letting go of his decision-maker role. After the horror stories I heard in rehab, don't think for a second I didn't realize how blessed I was to have him. While I was in ICU, Carrie even wrote the following in her first journal entry:

You collapsed on Monday and your superhero husband basically—no, not basically...exactly—saved your life.

Not many people can claim their spouse saved their life, can they? If he hadn't come home early from work that day, if he hadn't dialed 911 so quickly...the thought makes me shudder.

The role of caregiver and patient advocate was thrust upon him in a way he never expected when he signed on for this whole marriage thing. At least not for another fifty years or so. With this reality, our roles shifted organically, naturally. They had to. But when people get well again, no one ever talks about how hard it is to shift things back.

While I was in recovery, Paul became chief decision maker. He decided what we ate for dinner, since he cooked. He remembered all the doctors' instructions, since my memory was weak. He chose when we'd go out and when we'd stay in based on his schedule, since he drove.

Don't get me wrong: it was all with input from me. But my brain injury left me more indecisive than ever before. Deciding on a restaurant sent me into a tizzy. Making plans in advance taxed my organizational and prioritization damage. And any activity without Paul made me anxious and fearful of being alone.

As I got back into my life again and rebooted my business, I slowly clawed my independence back. Dipping my toe back into life again, I braved the bus on my own. I set coffee dates. I tackled client projects again. But at home, flipping those roles back to an equal partnership was not as easy as one would think.

Paul had gotten used to making choices for both of us. This had been okay with me for a while. But one night, my frustration boiled over and my patience ran out over something as simple as dinner.

"I'm in the mood for pasta with chicken for dinner. What do you think?" I suggested when Paul arrived through the front door.

"No need, baby. I already picked us up some tomato basil soup and a nice baguette from the market. I'll just make us a little salad and that'll be fine." He unloaded the grocery bags in the kitchen.

I blinked back tears as I watched him light the burner to heat up the soup.

"No. I want pasta with chicken," I said in a small but defiant voice.

"I'm sorry, I didn't know," Paul said. "I thought I was being helpful. We can have that tomorrow night if you want."

"No!" I screamed. "You went to the store and didn't even ask me what I wanted. You only thought about what *you* wanted to eat. Why don't I ever get a say? I'm not a child!" Proving otherwise, I stomped off to the couch and buried my face into a pillow, sobbing.

Paul was flabbergasted. Here he was, doing something nice for me. Something, quite frankly, most wives would love for their husbands to do for them. Confused and hurt, he wasn't sure what to say next.

"I just feel like I have no say in any decisions anymore," I told him after I'd calmed down.

"I'm sorry," he said, taking my hand as we sat next to each other on the couch. "I just got so used to handling it all on my own, I guess I've been on autopilot. For so many months, you've been indecisive or recovering and I'm just having a hard time adjusting back."

"I know and I appreciate that so much," I said, giving his hand a squeeze in return. "But I've got to start having a voice again, too. For my own sanity, if anything else."

It would have been so easy to let him continue making decisions and protecting me. Even though I was making great strides with picking up my life where it had left off, I was scared to be outside of the house, which was my comfort zone. As an extrovert and social animal, the fact that I was afraid in the first place scared me even more. I had never been a fearful person.

Part of the fear was self-consciousness over my physical appearance, my shaved head, and my vision and cognitive insecurities. Would I blurt out something stupid now that my filter was not working like it used to? Would I miss that stair and land on my face in front of everyone? Part of the fear was that I couldn't keep up with conversations as quickly as I used to. I couldn't deal with all the lights, crowds and sounds coming at me in a noisy bar or a crowded auditorium.

Who was this timid, fearful person inside of me? I had performed on stage, for Pete's sake. I mugged for TV commercials as a kid. Public speaking and workshops were a thrill for me. Walking into networking events where I didn't know a soul was easy as pie. Witty banter and a well-timed zinger in a fast-paced conversation were like champagne for breakfast, giving me a zippy little high.

Now I was different. My friends noticed that I was quieter among groups. I sat and watched the repartee from the sidelines because I wasn't quick enough to jump in with a sly comeback anymore.

I'd had enough.

I couldn't stand it anymore. If I was ever going to get my life back, there was no other solution except to face the fear. Head on. Gloves raised. A glint in my eye. Play chicken and stare it down until it melted into oblivion.

I couldn't live like a hermit and enjoy the life I was given a second chance at enjoying if I stayed on the couch with my dog. That would be like smacking God in the face for this miracle I'd been handed on a silver platter.

If I was ever going to figure out why I'd been spared, why I of all people was given a second, third and even fourth chance after all the bullets I'd dodged, I wasn't going to find the answer in my house. I had to find it *out there.*

What does it really mean to face the fear?

It means tenuously making plans even though you don't feel like it, or quickly agreeing to them before you're too chicken to back out.

So I forced myself to continue going out. I forced myself to keep going to book club every month and hanging out with the girls, buying the books on audio tape if needed. I forced myself to set a few coffee dates a week and not use my inability to drive as an excuse—there's a coffee shop about a minute's walk from my house, so I asked friends and even potential clients to meet me there. For the sake of my business, I forced myself to dip my toe back into the networking waters and attended workshops and mixers, supported all the way by friends who chauffeured me, held my arm in the dark to guide me, or read the small print on programs to me.

Was I petrified? Absolutely. Every outing took all the energy that my fatigued body and mind could muster. But I'm an actress, after all, so I used those acting chops to my advantage. I figured if I just plastered a smile on my face, got on with it and kept *acting* brave, and plunging myself into the icy water over and over again, eventually I'd start *feeling* brave again.

The goal was clear: regain my social mojo. Right or wrong, the approach I always take is to scratch an itch, not ignore it. That's what I did.

And then came the breakthrough.

On this particular balmy February evening in 2009, I had not quite gotten back to work and had yet to educate myself more fully in group rehab about what the heck was going on with me. Our friends Guy and Barb invited us to a happy hour goodbye party for a work colleague. Paul couldn't attend, but something inside me perked up and decided I should go. Without him. For the first time in months, my makeup and accessories called out, begging to be worn.

Barb and Guy agreed to pick me up and I felt like I was preparing for a date. I carefully applied my eye shadow and liner (which is tricky with vision in only one eye). My hair had recently been cut to even it up from the hack job that Mary and Paul had done in the hospital (bless them, but they are no stylists). As I recall, I dug out my unused and now sticky-nozzled hairspray to somewhat style my coif. Luckily, by this point, I was past the punk skinhead look and was sporting a bit more of a pixie-fresh vibe. The green sweater with the ruffled V-neck and a pair of designer jeans were simple yet polished. And then the pièce de résistance: Nancy's flower necklace completed my look.

Whoa. Accessories? *Are you kidding me?*

Alert the media.

As I appraised my work in the mirror that night, I stared at my reflection. The V-neck revealed the barely-visible tube of my shunt as it snaked from behind my ear and down the front of my still bony chest. Seeing it there, underneath my now made-up—and, to be honest, foreign-looking face—a burst of pride distracted me from the paralyzing fear.

Look at me, the tube shouted. Six months ago you were lying in an ICU ward and fighting for your life. Your hair may now cover your head scars, but every time you see me and that scar on your belly, you will never forget what a survivor you are.

I was still quiet but vibrating with anticipation when Barb and Guy picked me up, and we made it to the bar. Upon entering, I hooked my arm in Barb's, as we'd done so often in the last few months and she guided me up the stairs into the casual pub. I'm not sure I was ever so happy to smell stale beer in my life. Some friends who had heard my story but had not seen me since it all went down embraced me warmly.

You look terrific!

How are you feeling?

I can't believe what you've been through!

I stood close to Barb but felt the rush of a teenager who had just sneaked off to a party. Flushed with excitement, I was thrilled to be out and about again—on my own, without Paul.

"I'd love a vodka and tonic!" I practically screamed at the waiter, like a twenty-one-year-old on her birthday. Yup. Alcohol was allowed in small doses, but my tolerance was shot from so many dry months. One was all I needed.

I've done it, I thought to myself, bursting with shock and glee. The Old Me seemed to peek out from under the covers for the first time in a long time.

My ability to keep up with the conversation, to find the right words and unleash deadly zingers returned for the most part over the longer term—

or so I like to think. You'd have to ask others if I am really that witty and interesting.

Tired but walking on air, I bounded up the stairs into our family room. Paul was waiting.

"How was it?" he asked hesitantly.

"It was fantastic!" I cried. "I did it. I finally faked myself out enough to conquer my fear and feel like myself again!"

Paul breathed a sigh of relief. He had his own fears to face as well but they were psychological. He constantly worried about me feeling badly about myself. That's why he made so many of the decisions: he wanted to save my fragile psyche from any stress, friction or worry. Paul was never really concerned about my physical safety, per se. The day I first took the bus on my own, he made me practice calling his cell phone in case I needed help, but he knew I could handle myself out in the world and that I would ask for help if needed.

What broke his heart was how badly I felt about myself and my abilities when forced to confront the New Me. Almost like a parent, his biggest fear was that my confidence would be shaken and that there was absolutely nothing he could do about it. The evening was a win for him as well, since he knew I could get back out there without him—and without falling apart emotionally or coming home more self-conscious than when I had left.

Mind you, it wasn't all wine and roses after that. But it was a sure sign of progress. This tiny victory was the catalyst for getting back to email and work, proactively reconnecting with family and friends by phone, and in June 2009, getting back behind the wheel of a car.

Amazingly, I didn't need to take a test to do so, and perhaps the State of Washington would be none too pleased to learn a brain injury patient with vision problems had self-diagnosed herself enough to make this call. But I'm a smart cookie and there was no way I was going to endanger anyone's life, including my own.

That is why on a sunny Saturday in June, Paul drove me to Redmond so I could practice in the secluded safety of a Microsoft campus parking lot. If things went south, the only victim might be a squirrel. Or a landscaped median.

Face the fear. Face the fear. Face the fear.

Paul slid the car into park and opened his door to come around to my side.

"You're up," he said.

I'd waited so long for this and now it was here. Sliding into the left side of the car for the first time in about ten months was surreal. The seat belt felt funny on the other side of my body. It was like the first time I drove as a teenager. I actually checked all my mirrors and made my adjustments, just as my old driving instructors had taught me to do way back when.

Eyes wide and heart racing, I slid the car into drive and slowly took my foot off the brake. Flashbacks to eleven-year-old me backing the car out of the driveway under my father's watchful gaze came flooding back. Staring intently at the road without a single blink, I cruised at about ten miles an hour, eagerly searching from left to right until my eyes once again got used to scanning the road as they always had when driving. Practically, I wanted to make sure I had full use of my peripheral vision, as that had been one of the areas that the neuropsych test found a bit lacking. But that was over seven months ago, and by this time, I had my contact lens in my left eye and almost fully cleared sight in my right.

After about five minutes, I felt like I always had behind the wheel and giggled with relief. It really was like riding a bike. You know that joyful sense of freedom you felt when you first got your driver's license? Yeah, it was kind of like that.

Take that, Fear.

Coddling and reassurance had worked for the early days of my recovery. But eventually that can just turn into your own prison as you hide from the world. Sometimes it's better to face the fear head-on, over and over, and talk the talk until you finally relearn how to walk the walk.

Fake it until you make it, baby. It's painful but it works.

BUCKET LISTS

AUGUST 4, 2009.

The one-year anniversary of my aneurysm and brain hemorrhage rolled around faster—and yet, slower—than I ever would have thought possible. In some ways, it felt like I'd just been lying in the hospital bed, sightless, shorn and scared. On the other hand, if you had just met me, my hair was growing back in and my coloring (and weight) had returned to normal, so you would never have known the trauma I'd been through just one year earlier. Many of the scars were now on the inside, not the outside.

How does one celebrate (is that even the right word?) the day you almost died? Granted, I had avoided philosophical melodrama for most of the year as I focused on healing, while those around me looked to me as some kind of shaman who'd had a life-changing epiphany.

The truth is that, at the time, I didn't. Not really.

I was trying so hard to get back to normal that I couldn't stop to think about any greater cosmic significance.

But as the one-year anniversary rolled around—as I got back into my life, as my business picked up, as I started traveling to visit friends and take vacations again—this quest for significance grew stronger. I'm sure experts might say that means my healing was coming to an end.

Those who know me know I'm not much into the psychobabble. While I enjoy self-actualization, goal setting and even my religious faith as much as the next guy, I have a bit more trouble dwelling on my situation when I saw so many people in rehab who were much, much worse off. People who couldn't fully speak or walk or get back to work. Those whose family or friends had abandoned them because they could not deal with the new person they had become. It was heartbreaking and humbling all at the same time.

The night before the one-year mark, Paul and I enjoyed a romantic dinner out and a few glasses of wine to mark the occasion. Afterwards, in my bed, I sat wide awake and pondered the duality of "Wow! It's been a whole year since it happened" against "Wow! It's only been a year and look at all we've been through!" Amazing how time and space can morph to be as long or as short as you want them to be.

It seems "bucket lists" are all the rage these days, and the trend cropped up even more in the year following my aneurysm. Coincidence?

I'm not sure if this term had been around for a while or debuted with the Jack Nicholson/Morgan Freeman film of the same title. Regardless, it kind of irks me that it is swirling around everywhere, like shallow buzz about the latest hot handbag or must-have designer. While I love self-help and motivational goal-setting as much as the next gal (yes, I read Eckhart Tolle, so back off), I'm always leery when it takes the form of a blind fad. Shouldn't those themes be much more consistent and ongoing throughout our lives?

As the one-year anniversary of my brain hemorrhage passed, I was still trying to figure out what it all meant—and if it really meant anything anyway. Successfully distancing myself from the immediate recovery of the event—which was all about getting back to daily living—I entered this second phase of more thoughtful contemplation around the whole thing. Why did I survive? Why is my recovery going so much more miraculously than someone who has three children relying on her? If it was not "my time" yet, than what the heck is it I was meant to do here? What am I not finished with?

Small questions these are not.

Answers abound. Paul, who truly understands how lucky we are but is not a spiritual guy, will tell you, "This happened due to the genetics of a combination of weak vessels and high blood pressure that runs in the family. You are okay now because we got you to the hospital in time and the doctors were amazingly skilled. End of story."

Or maybe it's just as simple as what a sassy old friend of mine said when we met up for dinner after not seeing each other in person for over ten years. She had followed my story and progress through our online journal and social media updates and was dying to catch up with me. Her playful theory? "Maybe you are still here so that on this night, in this city, we could catch up over dinner and you can entertain and inspire me." I kind of like that answer.

Which brings me back to bucket lists. I feel in today's renaissance of enlightenment, we are just putting too much darn pressure on ourselves to "live our best life." I am all about going after what you want, not waiting, and experiencing all you can experience. But in my life, the adventures have happened pretty organically.

Sure, goals are great things. But when they start to consume you, to make you feel like you are less of a person if you don't accomplish them, that's where I have a problem.

My recovery was all about being gentle with myself, setting realistic goals, and not overwhelming myself with too much. I think this is a good way to live, brain injury or not. So rather than some of the more lofty bucket lists out there that seem to taunt and stress many of us—and make us feel like we are not doing, being, or seeing enough—mine became **a simple bucket list:**

1. Ensure you have at least one person in your life who understands you, accepts you for who you are and who makes you laugh. Just one will do. It could be a lover, parent, sibling or friend. If you don't have someone like this in your life, make it your mission to find him or her.
2. Spend at least one night of your life falling asleep to, and waking up to, the ocean. Wherever that might be.
3. Next time you are on a plane, bus or train with a rambunctious toddler or fussy baby, try to make the child smile. Just once. See how it makes you feel.
4. Call one long-distance friend a week. Not email. *Phone.* If you can't call, write a handwritten note.
5. Adopt a pet once in your life and give it a happy, loving home.
6. Say thank you to every bus driver or cabbie when you get off the bus or out of the cab. You never know how much that might turn around a bad day for them.
7. Once a day, ask one clerk, be it barista or cashier, "How are you doing today?"
8. Have one dinner outside on a warm summer night with friends, wine, candles and great conversation.

9. Each time you talk to a family member or a close friend, say "I love you" at the end of the conversation. You never know if it might be the last time.

10. Every year, make one trip to a place you've never been or somewhere out of your comfort zone. This could be another city in your own country, a foreign country, or it could be based on accommodations: if you are a hotel person, go camping. Try it for perspective.

My injury forced me to slow down and focus on the moment. It was not just a Hallmark card platitude, but a necessity. My goals became much less lofty but much sweeter.

I wrote a blog post musing about these thoughts shortly after my one-year anniversary. A dear friend of mine in San Francisco read this post. As I read her lovely emailed reply, I got the wind knocked right out of me and tears sprang to my eyes. It was titled, "I hesitated..." and it went a little something like this:

...to send you a note on your one-year anniversary. How do you celebrate someone not dying? So I waited and tried to figure out what to write. Thinking if maybe I just let it slip by, that would be the best thing. But then I finally summoned the courage to read your 365-day blog and, of course, found myself crying uncontrollably...to the point that both my husband and mother-in-law came over to find out what was wrong or who had died.

And I was like, no, someone lived! Try to explain that one!

Anyway, I just wanted you to know how much I admire you. Your strength and conviction. We always say, "No one but Maria could have persevered," and I truly believe this.

Thank you for being my friend and someone I look up to. I oftentimes think, "What would Maria do in this situation?" and so often, if I put my Maria Hat on, I come up with the right answer.

Holy smokes. She looks up to *me?*

See what I mean? Sometimes tragedy is a gift. I got my visit from the Ghosts of Christmas Past, Present and Future and attended my own funeral, in a way. My whole life, I just wanted to inspire, to make a difference, to matter. Who knew my brain had to literally explode for me to realize that the thousand tiny moments, interactions and love that you show people each and every day can add up to such a lasting impression? I always thought I was missing the big stuff: the grand gesture, the saving thousands of lives in Africa and, therefore, my life lacked real substance and meaning. It turns out you can touch the lives in your own backyard more profoundly than you think.

That is what I mean by a gift. And my hope for anyone reading this is that you don't need to suffer a traumatic brain aneurysm to realize how your little gestures and selfless acts matter to the world. Every bit of energy you put out there matters to someone, somewhere, sometime.

CLIMBING FOR THOSE WHO CAN'T

SLIGHTLY ANNOYED THAT my entire family and best friends had all been in Seattle immediately after my brain exploded, and that I could neither enjoy their company nor host them properly, I urged many of them to come back to visit the following summer in 2009.

My steadfast brother, Michael, who had already made two trips out here during the whole ordeal, was game and flew out for several July festivities. I was determined to show him more of beautiful Seattle than just the inside of an ICU.

The three of us—Paul, Michael and I—dropped Eddie off at doggie day care one jewel of a sunny day and drove a few hours to Mt. Rainier. Etched in the distance like some sort of movie set backdrop, Rainier is an awesome slice of raw nature juxtaposed next to the urban Seattle skyline. It looks much closer to the city than it is.

I had slowly started working out again. First, yoga a few times a week and of course I continued my Eddie walks. I was fighting through daily fatigue, which doctors had said could last up to a few years. But exercise did make me feel a bit better—even if only so my clothes fit better. Where initially my body swam in what had been my tight jeans, it didn't take long for things to catch up, especially with a more sedentary lifestyle. Hiking Mt. Rainer had been on our list for some time, and this was the perfect outdoor activity to share with my brother.

Paul scoped out an easy hiking trail near Paradise, a gorgeous little spot tucked into the south slope of Mt. Rainier's National Park. Wildflowers, glaciers and epic vistas await awestruck visitors as they wind up the sometimes steep trails.

The picture-perfect day gave us clear skies, comfortably warm temperatures and the clean, cool scent of flowers drifting toward us, as if distilled by pure ice.

My brother and I made quite a pair. Me, with my still healing stamina and increasing strength and he, just out of a brace from his ACL surgery. An easy trail was definitely in order to test both of our spirits.

We climbed. Passing teens in flip flops, we felt confident we could handle this trail. It wound around the mountain to a sweeping view of the valley and we had to stop every so often just to take it all in. Rolling fields of green dotted with color were occasionally interrupted by solid sheets of ice frozen in mid-roll down the mountain.

We took things slow, but then the trail went wonky. We were in shorts and sneakers, but hit some solid patches of ice and snow, forcing us to traverse on all fours in some places. Still seeing people in flip flops, I worried a bit but not too much.

However, as we wound up harder and harder terrain, I needed more time to catch my breath and Michael needed to ensure he didn't tweak his knee. Doubting that we were on the easy trail any more, Paul consulted signs and the map as we trudged onwards.

Finally, after over an hour and a half, we were still extremely high up the mountain on a trail that should have taken us thirty minutes to complete round-trip. I was losing steam, Michael's knee began to throb and we almost both viciously turned on Paul.

We finally passed a sign.

"Oh, we're on the wrong trail," Paul said. "We somehow ended up on the difficult one. How the hell did that happen?"

While a bit miffed, I swelled with pride. We had been on a difficult trail and, despite my health status, I had done it! Chalk one up for getting my exercise mojo back again.

As we rested before snaking our way back down, I enjoyed this perfect place of reflection. The beauty of everything for which I had to live—and be thankful—was all around me. Here I was, less than one year after surviving a massive brain hemorrhage and I had hiked a difficult trail at Mt. Rainier. This arduous hike up the mountain was a literal reflection of my journey thus far, and I'd done it. I was still here.

My body could physically carry me up the mountain. My eyes could take in the sweeping scenery. Once again, I felt a small twinge of guilt over those I had met who could never do something like this again. I was tired and my body had been stretched to its limit, but I was able to do it.

Was I doing it for them? I'm not sure. But nothing will get your body in motion faster than the fact that, but for a millimeter left or right on my artery, or a five-minute traffic delay for the ambulance, things could have turned out quite differently.

Sometimes that thought is too much to bear. Sometimes I think my head may literally explode again from trying to get my arms around that cosmic concept.

When the hectic and meticulously packed suitcase of your life gets dumped out all over the floor, it's actually a blessing. You can repack it however you want.

I'm a purger. Every few months, I get possessed by the ghost of some organizational demon and I clean out closets and empty drawers. With a vengeance. Maybe it's my type A personality again, but there is nothing as satisfying to me as when I stop shoving more things into a cramped closet and *start over*. I yank everything out and for a while, I bathe in the panic of my life's relics strewn all over the bedroom/office/hallway floor. But I love that fresh, airy feeling of being able to restructure the closet to be exactly what I need it to be. For a while at least, everything is organized, accessible and neat. And I've shed unwanted weight from my life with a quick trip to Goodwill.

My brain aneurysm was kind of like that.

My life had whipped itself up in a frenzy of change and stress until my head (quite literally) exploded. Once the rubble was cleared away, I saw the world in sharp focus.

My dirty little secret about this whole time in my life was that I actually think I prayed for this to happen. When I was starting the business, trying to make new friends, getting to know my way around the city, overwhelmed with doing things for the house, networking, getting my accounting systems in place—and all the while working with a coach and devouring self-help books to figure out what I really wanted to do with my life—I actually fantasized about getting sick.

Have you ever done that? Not that I wanted to be sick: I was just exhausted and wanted an excusable break from it all. I remember having many talks with Becky during that early time in Seattle, about how lost and overwhelmed I was.

"Maria, you have always been pretty adaptable to change," she said. "But I think with everything you've taken on this year, even you've hit your limit."

That was exactly how I felt. My threshold for change was really high but my cup runneth over—in a bad way. Maybe the only acceptable way to stop the madness and justifiably jump off the merry-go-round was to be stuck in bed. No one could blame me if that happened!

Believe me, the guilt of this unexpressed desire still hangs with me.

Now, I can clearly see that, for a while after the injury, my life was clean, pure and breathable. There was *space*. All the weeds had been pulled away, leaving a blank landscape upon which to replant.

I slowly began to fill it up again, as I do with the empty closet space, in exactly the way I wanted—in the way that would work best for me. What did I need to keep and what did I need to take to Goodwill?

Friends, family, connections, healing, peace, serenity, focus. Those were the things I chose to keep.

Competitiveness, perfectionism, caring about what others thought of me, and using society's borrowed definition of success—those were the things I chose to let fall away.

Don't get me wrong. There were tiny little setbacks all along the way. And the reality is that life has eventually become muddled and over-packed with crap again. But I'm more aware of it now. I stop and try to smell the roses a bit more often than before. And I can laugh at myself when I start to spin out of control. I valiantly cling to the lessons I learned during recovery as I don't want to let this newfound perspective just vanish into thin air.

So I eventually got off my ass during that first year back and got to work.

Years before, I had come up with an idea to write a heartwarming and humorous memoir about growing up Italian-American. Sort of like a *Sex and the City* meets *My Big Fat Greek* (Italian?) *Wedding*. I had dabbled with it here and there over the years, and had actually started writing some chapters before the aneurysm hit.

Now, I was bold. I didn't care about the right way to do things anymore. So I pitched a few agents and editors with my quirky idea. One publisher was interested. *Send me your book proposal,* her email said.

Crap. What's a book proposal?

Better figure it out, kid.

Without missing a beat, my good friend, Whitney—a bubbly and ambitious marketing consultant herself—told me about a class she was starting on how to write a non-fiction book proposal. I signed up that day and started the following week.

I tore through writing that proposal. Being in a class provided the structure that my New Brain needed to actually break it up into chunks and get it done. By late spring, I put the finishing touches on a lovely little proposal to send to the publisher. Whitney also invited me to join her and another gal in an informal writer's group to keep the momentum going and to share resources.

This group helped me maintain my newfound "Just do it!" attitude I so desperately wanted to hold onto out of this whole experience. We cheered each other on and when that first publisher said no, I thought, "What the hell? I now have this great proposal all done!" More agent and editor pitches followed and I just kept knocking them off my list.

At the same time, we encouraged each other to pitch our writing to magazines, just to get published articles and buzz through various channels. The year prior, just after being released from the hospital, someone had suggested, "You should totally write a book about your story." I had blanched at this. I was so not ready.

But maybe, after all I'd seen and been through in the last year, I could pitch a small story about the shocking effects of brain injury. Just an article. Maybe that was what I was meant to be doing, why I had survived.

I began to feel a huge sense of responsibility to share everything I'd learned and to be the voice for all those folks in rehab. Could that be why I was still here?

Maybe if I wrote about it, other people could avoid the destroyed relationships like those I had seen fellow patients experience. If only people knew what brain injury felt like and what it did to someone who otherwise looked fine, they'd be better equipped to handle it. They'd be more understanding.

Besides, getting more press would be good as I built my author platform, as it's called, for the memoir, I thought.

Bravely, I pitched my story idea to a few women's magazines, websites and even some TV and radio news programs. Rejection followed rejection. But again, I didn't care. I just kept hacking away at my list.

But then...a nibble. And another one. And a few more.

A few internet radio shows targeting women showed interest in my story. Pulling the microphone closer to me at the studio of one of them, I was relieved that the tone was light and uplifting. That was how I wanted the story told, I thought. Laughter had gotten me through so much of the past year, and I wanted to educate without maudlin melodrama.

Next, I received an email response from the producer of a local public radio show called *KUOW Presents*. He was intrigued by my story and wanted to speak to me about it before deciding to put it on the air.

Seriously? The local National Public Radio (NPR) affiliate radio station wanted to talk to *me*? I was overjoyed and petrified at the same time.

Whitney, the PR expert, coached me on how to deal with the call. I'm pretty media savvy and have dealt with the press in many previous jobs, but this was personal.

"He just wants to make sure you can speak intelligently and you're not crazy," she advised. "Make sure you have your main points written down and just be your charming self! You'll be fine."

I was not so sure.

With my brain injury, the biggest hurdle would be rambling on and on or forgetting my words. I had to remember to speak in sound bites and to be clear and consistent. The producer and I had a great chat, laughing at some of my crazier experiences, and we even hashed out several angles. He told me he'd be in touch.

Days later, he emailed me back and said that his boss had approved the segment and asked if I could be at the studio next week.

Um...hell, yeah.

And so it was that I sat in a quiet studio, just me and the producer, and I spoke candidly about what had happened and what I'd been through. Afterward, he shook my hand and told me it was great. It would air on Sunday, he said.

Riding in the car with Paul that Sunday, we flipped the station on. I heard my own voice come back at me and we both laughed. I was relieved that I sounded brave, coherent and natural. I'd acted on stage and screen for a long time, but this was different. This was about educating—and this was not a character, it was me. Who was this woman I heard coming through the radio who sounded so confident and sure?

The radio station posted a link to my personal blog, where I'd written some posts about my experience, including links to such resources as the University of Washington Medical Center, Wikipedia, the Brain Injury Association of Washington—and even my trusted Lumosity.

Emails arrived from people who had heard my show, and they thanked me profusely for sharing my story. I cried over many of these notes, especially those from people who'd been brain injured years ago and whose lives had been turned upside down by it. Such comments as "What you said about getting overwhelmed all the time? That's exactly how I feel!" were way too common.

One day a few weeks later, the phone rang in my home office. I don't have caller ID, so I picked it up.

"Hello, is this Maria Ross, who did the KUOW interview a few weeks ago?" "Yes, it is," I said with some trepidation. "Who is calling and how can I help you? This is my office number."

"Please excuse my interruption," the woman on the other end said. "I harassed the folks at the radio station until they finally directed me to your website and I found your office number. My name is Judy and my son was brain injured years ago in a car accident. He's twenty-seven and still needs to live at home."

"Oh, I'm so sorry, Judy. But how can I help you?"

"Well, your experience was so enlightening. What you described is so much of what he goes through every day. I've been searching for so many resources and can't really find any good ones. Can you recommend any for us?"

My spidey-sense warned me to tread carefully here. I reminded her that I am not a medical doctor and that she should consult with her physician, because I knew nothing about her son's case.

"Oh, I don't mean medical resources. I just mean what personally or emotionally worked for you to get back on your feet again. Please. Anything you can direct me to would be helpful." Her voice cracked from what sounded like a long journey of desperation.

"Sure, I can tell you what I found and what worked for me, Judy." I gave her some websites and told her about my in-home therapies and UW Medicine's amazing rehab programs. I also told her about books I had investigated, such as *My Stroke of Insight* by Jill Bolte Taylor. And, of course, Lumosity, for the brain games.

"Thank you so much for sharing all of this with me," she said. I could tell right then and there that I was blessed to have had the resources and expertise all around me at UW Medicine. Some people are not as lucky.

The realization hit me that, no matter what, the aneurysm in my brain had probably been going to burst at some point. It had been forming and growing for a while before that fateful August day in 2008, I'm sure, and it had only been a matter of time. So what good deed had I done in another life to be in this city, close enough to this hospital, with these resources all around me?

172 ... MARIA ROSS

The difference between life or death—and healthy recovery or endless frustration—can hang on the same thing that sells real estate: location.

I was lucky. Judy's son was not. What a sobering thought.

Our writing group soldiered on, encouraged by several small victories. I added the NPR media appearance to my proposal. When my friend found a possible agent for her book, I pitched the same woman about my memoir idea.

"Memoirs are tough," she said. "We're actually looking for interesting and innovative books about business or marketing."

A light bulb flashed above my head.

"Really? Well, I'm not sure if you're interested, but I have this little fifteen-page e-book I created about branding for small businesses. Would you be interested in seeing it?"

Opportunity knocked, and without fear, I invited him in.

Keep in mind that my fear was bi-polar. I could be fearless about opportunities, saying what I thought and going after what I wanted. But I was still afraid of all the little things I've mentioned in the previous pages that I had to deal with during my recovery.

It was an odd duality that even I couldn't reconcile.

But the confidence from more tangible actions, such as pursuing the book opportunity with this agent, leaked into the psychological and emotional areas. Being brave about things that, in my mind, didn't really matter made it easier to be brave about things that did matter.

The agent loved my e-book and asked if I was interested in having her husband's new small press be the publisher. I couldn't believe it! Butterflies fluttered in my stomach as I realized that I had the chance to become a published author. Dreaming of this since I was six years old and writing fantastical stories about mice families, I hadn't quite envisioned a business book as my first opus. But there it was—an opportunity to turn lead into gold.

As I mentioned, had I not been in recovery from my brain injury and had the time—and the need—to write the e-book, I would have had nothing to re-pitch the agent. But life is funny that way, isn't it?

I signed the publishing contract by Christmas and, for the next four months, banged out the manuscript. Putting all my branding and marketing knowledge down on paper was actually a great way to get more fully back into my work groove.

And that is how, just a year and a half after almost dying, I realized one of my life's dreams by writing a book. Paul said a few words at my book launch party held at a funky little bar and bistro in Seattle. My darling Carrie actually got her butt on a plane and flew in to be at my side once again. Love her.

In front of the now smiling faces of friends, work colleagues and clients, Paul made this business accomplishment personal.

"Many of you know what Maria's been through this past year and a half. I'm so immensely proud of her for all she's accomplished in that short period of time. After her brain aneurysm, she had memory, vocabulary and even physical troubles. And now here she is a published author. I'm so proud of my wife."

Those who came expecting just a dry talk on branding and marketing may have wiped away a tear or two, I'm sure.

This moment was not about business success, but rather the resiliency of our spirits to bounce back no matter how many times we fall—and to come back stronger, fiercer and, in an odd twist, more humble and open at the same time.

PART FOUR

Life Reframed

I have at times been wildly, despairingly, acutely miserable, but through it all I still know quite certainly that just to be alive is a grand thing.

\- Agatha Christie

Adversity is like a strong wind. It tears away from us all but the things that cannot be torn, so that we see ourselves as we really are.

\- Antoine Marie Roger de Saint-Exupery

TWO LONG YEARS

AUGUST 4, 2010. The two-year anniversary. What a crazy two years it had been.

My business was booming with two big clients and good money coming in the door. Although I still struggled with prioritization and memory, I was handling things much better than I had been. I constantly went back to the memory, focus and emotional strategies I'd learned in rehab to cope with all the work. Every now and then, I made mistakes but my trusted colleagues knew my situation and helped me out by remembering details of phone conversations or action steps. The year 2010 proved to be a banner financial year for my business, going from nearly nothing in 2009 to six figures in revenue. My accountant was duly impressed.

The branding book was doing extremely well, and seeing positive customer reviews pop up on Amazon was like Christmas morning. Emails flew across my computer from all over the country—and even the world—from entrepreneurs and small business owners everywhere, thanking me for the simple lessons and "practical yet entertaining advice."

Wow! I was helping many people live their entrepreneurial dreams and support their families. It warmed my heart to no end.

And, joy of joys, *my hair had grown back!* Oh, come on, I'm a chick. Little things like this mean a lot. I will always feel the hard ridge in my skull from the shunt, but by this time, it was finally hidden under rows of curls.

But back to the two-year anniversary. To answer the question I know you have, yes, I will remember August 4 for the rest of my life. Well, the

178 ... MARIA ROSS

date anyway. As mentioned, I don't recall the actual day at all, nor most of the ensuing month in ICU.

That night, Paul and I went to dinner to celebrate life, luck, blessings and joy. While running errands the weekend prior and enjoying our warm Seattle summer, I had said to Paul, "You know, it'll have been two years on Wednesday. I think we should go out to dinner to celebrate."

I was touched that he didn't even hesitate.

"Yes," he said, "let's definitely do that."

On Tuesday, the day before our dinner date, I had a follow-up appointment with my retinal surgeon, Dr. Kinyoun. While I religiously saw him every six weeks for almost the first year, it had been about a year since our last meeting. His office had moved from its prior location at University of Washington Medical Center back to a brand-new building near where the whole saga had begun: Harborview Medical Center.

We greeted each other warmly.

"Good to see you looking so well!" he said. He had never seen me with long curly hair, at my usual weight and or even with a healthy skin tone.

After his now familiar pokes and prods, he gave me an all-clear diagnosis on any issues left over from the Terson's. My right eye had re-absorbed about 99 percent of all the blood in the eye, leaving no more rose petals in my vision. My only issue now was the cataract in my left eye. Through regular monitoring, we knew it was holding steady.

I arrived to my appointment early and went to fetch a much-needed morning coffee from a building located across the street from the entrance to Harborview's emergency room. My gait slowed as I stared at the entrance.

Now, mind you, while I don't remember the ER at all, I shudder every time I walk by it because I think of Paul, all alone and lost in his fear and worry. It tears my heart into a thousand pieces. While I am spared that painful trauma of memory, he still cringes and gets quiet every time we're near a hospital or an ambulance races by.

I paused and watched the ER doors. Blessedly, there was not much going on that day. I thought of all the lives that are forever changed by that entrance. I could almost envision the ambulances racing in, the families aimlessly wandering around in shock, the countless people who lose their loved ones through that doorway each and every day. So much pain, so much loss.

But I had made it. Paul and I had made it. I had regained my vision, restored my strength, got back to my business—and even wrote a book, for goodness' sake. How far we'd come in two amazing years.

Did I come back wiser, more thankful, more aware? I like to think so. Even when stress takes over and I'm overwhelmed, I try to at least take a second and say aloud, "You're still here, Maria. Nothing else matters." And I breathe again.

So I went to my appointment and then drove home. Eddie greeted me like a rock star at the door, wiggling his butt, wagging his tail, doing his little happy dance and demanding attention as if nothing had ever happened in our lives.

Gotta love dogs.

Even though I had a ton of things to do, I left the computer off so I could snuggle with Eddie for a while, smile at the sun on the patio outside my office, and thank God for not being ready for me yet.

And then I went back to work.

W E HAVE A fond affection for Microsoft.

I don't care how much you love your damn iPhone or iPad. Microsoft's benefits absolutely rock. Their health care plan paid 100 percent of our bills—yeah, that's 1-0-0—with no co-pays. We even had an amazingly generous and organized case manager from the insurance company assigned to us who didn't make us lift a finger.

"I've never felt like a 'company guy' my entire career," Paul has said on more than one occasion, "but Microsoft paid for my wife's brain."

Yup. To the tune of...when the ICU stay, in-patient rehab, drugs, surgeries, in-home care and therapy, group outpatient therapies, neuropsych tests, prescriptions, follow-up visits to at least four or five doctors, eye surgeries, follow-up angiograms and MRIs, and anything else you can think of (including the $800 for a five-minute ambulance transfer between hospitals) are all factored in...over half a million dollars.

I know. We're the luckiest freaking people in the world. We would have been in serious trouble, if you also consider the fact that I hardly made any money the year following this whole mess.

This entire ordeal made me see health care in a whole new light. What would we have done if Paul's work hadn't paid for all of this? What if a homeless person has a brain aneurysm? Not once did we ever have to weigh treatments against cost. When the doctors said I needed something, Paul had to give medical consent as my spouse and was able to approve without hesitation. My heart aches for anyone who has to weigh such a choice just because of circumstances or a bank account balance. Who's to say my life is worth more than someone struggling to get by? No one.

I was lucky that our insurance plan also paid for the regular follow-up exams and scans required to monitor my situation. The aneurysm coil needed check-ups to ensure it still fit correctly. Plus, the emergency angiogram I had on that fateful August 2008 day revealed another tiny aneurysm in my brain, not too far from the first one. It was teeny tiny and nothing to worry about if I kept my blood pressure in check, but the neurosurgeon felt yearly scans would be the best way to keep an eye on everything. It turns out many people have aneurysms they don't know about—unless, like me, something bad happens to announce their existence.

About six months following my injury, I had my first follow-up angiogram to verify that the coil was secure and to check on the other, smaller aneurysm. I had been in that ward before but of course didn't remember a thing. Arriving bright and early that winter morning, I placed all my clothes in a plastic bag and donned my familiar hospital robe. Warm, toasty blankets staved off the chill in the air. Paul held my hand as I lay waiting for them to prep me for the procedure. A nurse pierced my arm to set up the IV tube for my wonderful calming drugs, as I thought of them. When they were ready for me, Paul gave me a quick kiss and headed off to work while they wheeled me into the angiography suite.

A lab-type room greeted me with a huge scanning machine attached to the ceiling. Three or four bustling residents and technicians kindly doted on me, making sure I was warm and comfortable. Pulling up my gown, they placed a modest little covering over my lady parts and prepped the groin area for the procedure. As they did this, the anesthesiologist talked me through what she would do.

"We're giving you some drugs that will not put you under completely but will make you calm and comfortable," she said. "I'll be right here the whole time in case you need more, but you will need to be aware enough to follow directions from us for the scan, okay?"

The drugs. Oh, the drugs. They were like a combination of valium and brandy and, while I was not completely knocked out, I instantly felt a slow warmth creeping like honey through my veins. It was like drinking three bottles of red wine—minus the hangover.

"I'm so warm and cozy," I purred amidst my other babbling. "That stuff is great. Can I have some to get me through the rest of the day?"

Um...no.

They began the angiogram by inserting a catheter in my groin and threading it up my femoral artery toward my brain, just like they had when I was in the ICU—but this time, I was aware of what they were doing and was a little bit freaked out. Fortunately, I didn't feel a thing. Slowly, they injected dye as I lay flat on the table. A bizarre x-ray-type camera floated all around me, taking 3-D pictures that look like spaghetti strands, I found out later. At times, I was asked to hold my breath or lay completely still so as not to blur the picture.

I'm not sure how long I lay there, but it was over fairly quickly. After carefully removing the catheter, a resident held a bandage to the wound and applied constant pressure for about fifteen to twenty minutes while we chitchatted about both of us being from the Midwest. Applying pressure is vital: bleeding from an artery is no laughing matter, so they must be sure the clotting process can start effectively and help avoid infection.

Whisking me up to recovery, the orderlies placed my bed back in the recovery room and my long day began. I was comfortably propped up on pillows but was not allowed to bend my right leg—the leg they used for the procedure—for eight hours. I had to keep it outstretched and as stable and still as possible so that the wound would clot completely.

Eight hours flat on your back with someone at your beck and call sounds divine...until your lower back starts aching, and you get bored with lying prone and watching bad daytime TV. The hours ticked by slowly as I eagerly awaited Paul's arrival around 5 p.m. to take me home.

A few days after the scan, I met with my neurosurgeon, a.k.a. my Brain Ninja, to discuss the results and ask any questions. Dr. Ghodke greeted Paul and me and happily shook our hands.

"Wow," he said. "Your recovery has been remarkable."

That first year, I was still frail and shorn, but I was a far sight better than when he'd seen me in the ER that fateful day. Even his resident, who had also been part of my trauma care, kept staring at me in disbelief because we were having such a normal conversation. Did I mention subarachnoid hemorrhages are pretty bad news?

And then Dr. Ghodke said something that utterly moved me:

"It's recoveries like yours that are the reason we go into medicine."

It sticks with me to this day.

In 2010, one year later, I had another follow-up angiogram and—dare I say—I understand why people can get addicted to painkillers and the like. When Paul came to pick me up that second time, a chocolate milkshake once again in hand as I'd requested, he half-joked that I should pipe down on the "drug love" or the medical staff was going to start getting worried.

These results showed the coil was holding well, and the other aneurysm had not grown. They were watching to ensure the neck of the aneurysm (similar to the neck of a balloon) didn't stretch too much from the coil, which would essentially make the opening so wide that it would render the coil useless in blocking the blood flow. That's why they make the coil out of platinum, because it's a softer metal that won't create too much stress from movement.

My follow-up exams were scheduled yearly. In 2011, the recovery-intensive, day-long angiogram was replaced by a mere Magnetic Resonance Angiogram (MRA), which is a type of the more familiar Magnetic Resonance Imaging (MRI) scan. An MRA can detect problems in the blood vessels that may be causing reduced blood flow. With an MRA, both the blood flow and the blood vessel walls can be seen. Unlike the regular angiogram, the MRA took less than an hour and, afterwards, I simply got dressed and went home.

I donned a cloth gown, lay flat on my back on a narrow table between foam blocks that kept my head perfectly still, and then was slid into a tube that took scans of my brain. If you watch *House* on TV, they do this every episode. This one was a zippy in-and-out process, although *sans* drugs. Bummer.

Because this was a MRA, our follow-up appointment with Dr. Ghodke was scheduled immediately after the procedure, rather than days later.

His colleague had handled the last year's checkup, so it'd been about two years since he'd seen me. I looked like the old Maria—and nothing like the shell he had seen. We had emailed in the interim, as I asked him if he'd be a source for me should my article idea get picked up by the media. He had generously agreed and told me I could ask him questions any time.

"You look fantastic!" he said. I smiled.

"Your results look good. The coil is holding well. Some slight stretching in the neck of the aneurysm, but it all looks fine. We'll just keep an eye on it, and we can always go in if we need to." He pulled the scans up on the computer and Paul and I tried to make sense of the spaghetti-like strands we saw on the screen.

"Thank God you can understand what you're seeing there, because I don't know how you'd find a tiny aneurysm in that mess," I said.

He laughed, "Well, we know what to look for."

He showed us scans from the day I had been brought into the ER and how they compared with the scans they had just taken. The August 2008 scan clearly showed the big mass on my brain vessel.

And the bright white halo of light surrounding my brain?

"That was all the blood," he said matter of factly.

Dr. Ghodke clicked the mouse a few more times for different perspectives and stopped on one image. He pointed to a tiny little bump along all the vessels that totally looked like it belonged there.

"And there it is, the other aneurysm. The size has not gotten bigger, which is great news."

Seriously? How in the hell did they know *that* was an aneurysm?

Actually, I don't care how. They just do. Bless them.

I love how Dr. Ghodke always takes the time to show us scans and explain what is going on in my brain. I itched to crack a sarcastic joke about him getting inside my head but Paul might have divorced me on grounds of cheesy humor.

"See this?" He pointed to one scan that showed a smudged-out black spot, less than one inch in diameter, in the front right center of my brain. It was like someone had erased part of the scan.

"That is your brain damage from the bleed," he said. "Those are dead brain cells."

Whoa.

I stared at the picture. There it was. Proof of my brain injury, lit up by the glow of the computer screen.

I felt...relieved.

While I was thankful for my miraculous recovery, I had struggled for two years with the emotional, psychological and cognitive effects of the brain injury. I had berated myself for not being able to do things the way I used to. I had cried in vain over why once-simple tasks proved difficult or overwhelming. I had questioned if my memory issues, my mental quickness and my multitasking losses were simply my imagination or were actual and real effects of what I'd experienced.

Brain injury is tough because you still have so much "there" there. In my case, it felt like just enough had been tampered with to drive me crazy... but I wasn't ever quite sure what, exactly, had been messed up. It's like coming back to your house and having the eerie sense that someone had been rifling through your things, but you can't quite put your finger on what was moved or disturbed. You just know something is off.

"I'm not crazy!" I thought. "There's a real reason why I still struggle with so much."

My unseen glitches had just been validated in one fell swoop.

Don't get me wrong. I was not happy to see the brain damage, but I was relieved that there was an explanation, a reason, for those tiny little hiccups I still experience on a daily basis.

I did indeed look fine on the outside, and I had come so far in such a short period of time, in the grand scheme of things. But I was not the one holding myself back. These daily issues were real and, no matter how far I'd come, it was now clear that the damage would never really go away.

This knowledge, this validation, was more liberating than I can ever express.

PART FIVE

———

Life Goes On

*I arise in the morning torn between a desire to improve the world and a
desire to enjoy the world. This makes it hard to plan the day.*

- E. B. White

*Life's challenges are not supposed to paralyze you; they're supposed
to help you discover who you are.*

- Bernice Johnson Reagon

GETTING BACK TO LIFE . . . AND THE BIG QUESTIONS

A<small>BOUT TWO YEARS</small> after my brain injury, I was driving down the street to a coffee meeting. It was sunny, and I sang along to some silly pop song on the radio, as I am prone to do when in a good mood. The trees were in glorious summertime bloom. As I drove down a shady street right near my house and fancied myself giving Taylor Swift a run for her money, I glanced over to the sidewalk.

Struggling with a walker, a focused young man slowly but surely made his way down the street. He heaved the walker forward a bit and then dragged his legs to keep up. Rinse and repeat. Rinse and repeat. You could tell his muscles would not do exactly what he wanted them to do, but, by God, he was going to make his way down that sidewalk.

Instantly, I thought of a young man in my rehab therapy group, a brilliant mathematician and programmer, who had had a brain tumor removed. I could still picture his wire-framed glasses, sandy brown hair, alert eyes and tenderhearted grin. Struggling to walk and talk—and using a walker similar to that of the man I had just seen on the street—the guy in my group had not lost his wry sense of humor as he struggled to deliver one-liners and entertain our merry band of brain misfits.

I quickly brought my gaze back to the road. Then I pulled over and burst into body-wracking sobs.

As the tears streamed down my cheeks, I raged at God for the first time. Not about my own situation being so bad, but rather about it being so good:

Why did you spare me? Huh? Why was that poor guy in our group destroyed but I'm fine, driving my car to stupid appointments and running meaningless errands? By the luck of the draw, I'm fine and that poor guy struggles to walk and talk and will never work again doing what he loves to do. What the hell makes me so special? No children are counting on me, no lives depend on me for survival, no one's world would fall apart if I was dead. Why am I still here, huh? Why the hell would you spare me from all that pain and yet ruin the lives of other, better people?

I sat down on the couch later that day and told Paul about the incident.

He was stricken. "You are my everything. You make me happy, you make me feel loved. You know who counts on you? *I do.* And so does Eddie."

Eddie perked up at the mention of his name, thinking there might be treats involved, but when he realized there was no food, he promptly sank back down into the couch cushion and went to sleep.

I couldn't help but laugh at the dog's reaction, which broke the tension.

Paul gave me the biggest hug you can imagine. "Don't ever say that you don't matter to anyone. You matter to me!"

These unexpected moments of survivor's guilt hit me pretty often, once the immediate recovery struggles and dangers had passed. They tended to pop up during the everyday moments of my life, like this one, when I had simply been driving down the street.

I've always tried to live a good life and to give back where I could, but I'm no Mother Teresa. I give money to charity and have given my time and talents to my church and various non-profits over the years.

But, surely, all of that did not make me worthy of getting this second chance, did it?

My philanthropic imperative, as I like to call it, had begun when I was in college. I found a volunteering pamphlet in my business school's career office. It talked about all the benefits of giving your time and energy to a worthwhile cause, to give back to the community. On the back, in big, bold, white letters, was written: *Volunteering is the rent you pay for the space you take.*

You can blame it on the Catholic guilt on which I was raised, if you like, but that concept has never left my mind since.

I was actually donating pro-bono marketing expertise to a local foster care and adoption agency when my aneurysm hit. I wasn't able to attend the final presentation, but my team members said it was a success and the agency was truly grateful.

All of that is well and good, but I'm certainly not the person who's cutting through welfare red tape, opening homeless shelters, doling out food at the soup kitchen every month or organizing charity drives to send blankets and food to earthquake victims. I'm the person who bends over backwards to *contribute* to those causes and spread the word, but I've never felt I was noble by any stretch of the imagination. And I have struggled with this idea of my calling, and what I actually give back to the world, for my entire life.

Oprah Winfrey has long been an idol of mine not because of her Favorite Things or her book club, but because she has adopted an attitude that with great blessings comes great responsibility. I strive to emulate that. Her words, deeds and financial support have changed countless lives. I could care less about her weight-loss struggles, fabulous wealth or controlling management style. Given all the good she has done in the world, if this woman wants to enjoy the spoils of her hard work and success with a Tuscan villa, a compliant staff, a manor house compound, or hell, even her own private airport for all I know, I say let her have it. She's earned it.

My brain injury and miraculous recovery brought all of those questions about my calling back into sharp focus. Sure, I gave back when I could. But I didn't feel I'd earned the extent of my good fortune. In fact, I felt like I hadn't done enough.

So why was I still here? And what could I do to live a life worthy of this second chance? I had to do even more.

A personal development coach once told me that you can actually damage yourself by doing good works for the wrong reasons. It's not healthy if you're doing them out of some sort of twisted obligation. She was right.

But at that point in my recovery, in my mind, it wasn't just about doing good things for others; it was about doing penance. I started volunteering with a vengeance, and Paul worried that I was back to my old tricks of over-committing and stressing out.

My chosen causes, however, all shared a common theme: using my voice to help others.

I joined my church choir, which I hadn't done since high school. While not quite the philanthropic effort, it was a way to get out in the community, give back to my church, and scratch my itch to perform.

I also signed up for volunteer training classes at the Seattle Animal Shelter. This was the wonderful place where we'd gotten our beloved Eddie, and after his vital role in my recovery, I wanted to give back. The shelter does fantastic, innovative work to help foster and adopt out homeless, abandoned and abused animals. Paul was worried that being there would

192 ... MARIA ROSS

add to my depression, but it's not a sad place at all. It's one full of love and warmth. I dabbled with volunteering for a few of their programs, but not quite finding the right fit. Eventually, I started donating my marketing expertise and helping them with a branding effort and a yearly auction. It felt good to not just talk about animal welfare anymore, but to somehow contribute to being the voice for those wonderful creatures who want nothing but to be loved.

But I needed to speak for humans as well. I felt I had a responsibility to be a voice for my fellow brain-injury patients. Talking is a gift I have (or a curse to those around me) and being an actress and a public presenter, I was in the perfect position to share what I'd learned about brain injury to educate others and to shed light on the patient experience. Others may have had their speech or memory impacted more severely than I did, but I could at least speak for them.

After seeing a flyer on one of my doctor's visits, I signed up to be a patient advisor at the University of Washington Medical Center. Serving on the patient and family education committee, I represent "the voice of the patient experience" and help with initiatives that put patients first. When someone dreams up a new manual or video for patients and their families, it's my job to sanity check it and remind everyone what a patient is thinking and feeling in the chaos of a hospital stay.

This work is my way of giving back to the amazing folks at this great hospital. I also speak about the patient perspective at new hire orientations. My message is that whether you are a doctor, or work in the billing department or serve coffee at the café, your actions make a difference to stressed and shell-shocked patients and their families.

In this patient-advisor role, I have also gotten the opportunity to share my personal experiences at orientation. I get to tell new hires what meant the most to me and my family during my stay and while I was in outpatient rehab.

I usually explain, "No matter what area of care you work in, you make a difference to the experience of a patient and their family. If you take appointments, you never know what the person on the other line has just been told about their father or sister. If you work in the café, you never know if the man you are serving was just told his wife is being rushed into emergency surgery or that she may never walk again. You have no idea what burdens they bear when they show up at your door. But you can choose to either lighten the load or add to the stress during that interaction."

My work at orientations got noticed, and I was asked to share my patient story and kick off a two-day leadership conference dedicated to the patient- and family-centered care philosophy. The conference planners wanted to remind the attendees representing various hospital departments that this training was more than a philosophy to which to pay lip service. It was about how everyone's role up and down the chain of command impacts real people and real lives. About 500 department heads, hospital leaders, doctors and administrative staff sat rapt as I told my story from the ballroom podium.

"You must remember that before we arrive in the ER, the OR, or show up as a patient in the hospital, we are people out there in the community, living our lives."

Intellectually, I think all medical practitioners know this, but it helps to remind them that we are more than the sum of our parts to be poked and prodded.

This is part of what you live with as a trauma survivor: The knowledge that people whose names you never knew and who you will never see again took care of you, worked frantically to stop your internal bleeding, comforted your family during a shocking nightmare, and performed a thousand small heroic actions that saved your life.

And you never get the chance to thank them.

I saw this as my chance.

Never underestimate the power of first-person experience in getting people to sit up and listen. While I spoke, you could have heard a pin drop. Much more nervous than I usually am when speaking, I had practiced my presentation for days because I knew I was representing more than myself during that speech. That day, I knew I was the voice of everyone in my rehab group.

Maybe this is why I'm still here, I thought. Maybe my role is to share this information and tell these stories and make things easier for those who have no voice.

Brain injury is not just about the physical aspect of how a person looks on the outside. It's not just about doctors being able to save our lives, but about understanding and empathizing with the internal struggles that brain injury patients have to deal with on a daily basis: the unseen battles, frustrations, self-doubt and loss of identity.

I was speaking to these attendees, but I felt like I was speaking to everyone out there, on behalf of those patients who don't know why they are struggling, or why they can't do what they used to do, or whose friends and families have abandoned them due to ignorance. In my small way, maybe I was helping them—or helping those who might come after them with the same issues and fears.

I wanted so badly to get this speech right, to strike a chord, to make an impact. I wrapped up my fifteen-minute talk with a final thought.

"Most of all, I want to say thank you. As a trauma patient, the one thing you have to live with is the fact that countless people whose names you will never know had a hand in saving your life and comforting your family. And that can be hard. So this is my chance to finally say thank you for the wonderful care you gave to me. And just remember that patient- and family-centered care matters just as much to us as patients and to our recovery as the medical prowess that you show every day."

The attendees broke their silence with thunderous applause and a standing ovation. As the director running the event handed me a colorful bouquet of wildflowers, he thanked me for sharing my story and reminding everyone why they were spending two days on this important topic. As I left the room, all I could see was that bright, physically damaged young man from rehab, with his eyes shining and his spirit unbroken by the hand he'd been dealt.

I fervently hoped that I had made him proud.

THE CHICKEN OR THE EGG

I'VE BEEN ASKED, "Do you think your brain defines who you are?"

Interesting question.

I've learned that our brain function is responsible for not just our physical being, but how we plan, whether we're organized or not, how much initiative we have, and whether we get angry, sad, happy or hopeful. It conducts each instrument that makes up the grand orchestra of who we are:

"He's a go-getter."
"She's a neat freak."
"She's good with numbers."
"He is such a spontaneous guy."

All of these personality types and traits that define us as human beings can be impacted by damage to our brains. If that happens, then who are we? Does brain function dictate your personality? Or, if you believe personality is a part of your soul, then does that come first? And if it does come first, does it dictate the way your brain learns to operate?

I can say from my experience that many definitions I had for myself no longer apply, now that I've had brain damage. I used to be much more of a neat freak, always tidying up and avoiding clutter. Now I let things slide a bit and Paul often has to step in. I used to be a master multitasker, able to juggle a full-time, demanding executive role while still making time for performing in plays, writing freelance articles, and having a pretty full social dance card. Now I must balance my time in chunks, leaving room for only one or two networking events per week or committing to only one big volunteer project every six months. I used to be a bit more spontaneous. I once dropped a boyfriend off at the airport and decided when I got there to simply hop the plane with him, buy a new outfit when I got to our destination, and call in sick. Now? Forget it! The thought alone gives me a headache.

And when confronted with too many decisions all at once, such as trying to book a round-trip flight online when there are dozens of time and cost options, I am literally paralyzed into silence and inaction. Paul has learned to recognize that look, that total my-internal-system-must-shut-down look, and he will gently offer to walk me through it one step at a time.

I still get overemotional at times, bursting into tears if my husband unexpectedly needs to work late and our dinner plans change, or tearfully hugging a confused Eddie when we randomly walk by the same Missing Dog poster we've seen fifty times. I'm much more sentimental than I used to be.

As for being overwhelmed, I'm learning to recognize the triggers and manage them. Crazy, chaotic scenes, like Times Square or a recent U2 concert, can cause a flurry of panic they never did before. Now I know that I just need to grab someone's arm, look down, shut out the noise and breathe deeply to steady myself again. And packing for a trip? There has been only one time recently when the overflow of tasks to remember and things to do didn't make me cry. But, hey, at least now we can joke about it.

My case is unique in that my life went through some major changes right before the brain injury. Many of the deltas that I face could be a result of the brain damage—or they could just be where I am in my life right now. I work from home alone most of the time, and not in a social office setting. I have a dog to think about when considering taking off at a moment's notice, I don't have a corporate structure to lean on that tells me what I need to do and how to prioritize my time. The fact is that I'm getting older, too. Who knows if I would still struggle with the overwhelm, the fatigue, mood swings or the memory lapses—brain injury or not?

In the end, I don't think the answer really matters. The fact is that I had a brain hemorrhage that almost killed me. If not for a divine (or lucky) set of circumstances, such as being at home when I collapsed and having my husband come home early that day, living a mere five miles from the four-state region's Level 1 trauma center that attracts some of the very best trauma surgeons from around the country, having access to one of the leading neural rehab programs in the country...if it weren't for these facts, things may have turned out very differently for me.

When someone hears my story, there's not a person who doesn't have a wife/brother/neighbor/teacher/daughter who has not been touched by brain injury—traumatic or not. This number has gone up in recent years as vets return home from the wars abroad. Sooner or later, brain injury will affect you. And given how little we know about its effects in our everyday lives, I foresee more pain and misunderstandings for those dealing with it, much like I saw in the lives of the people in my rehab group.

I've heard a few stories about people who "hit their heads pretty hard" when they were younger, and after hearing what I experienced, they said, "Oh, my God, that is exactly what my life has been like!" It's like they've unlocked an explanation for behaviors or emotions that have tormented them for years because they just didn't know what the heck was happening. Approximately 1.7 million people suffer a traumatic brain injury annually, with 52,000 people dying from the injury, but many of the survivors think they can just shake it off.[20]

In 2010 and 2011, many states passed a slew of laws to protect athletes from head injury. In many of these laws, coaches are required to undergo concussion training, and certain checkups and milestones must be met before an injured young athlete can get back into the game. I now have a new appreciation for these laws. Due to a particular young man's injury, Washington State became the first to adopt a Lystedt Law, which requires young athletes who've suffered concussions to get medical clearance before competing again. As a result, twenty-two other states have since adopted such a law and even the National Football League has raised awareness about concussions and player safety.

I also feel more strongly about using protective helmets. I had never skied with a helmet before (and used to mock Paul for doing so) but you can be sure that when I hit the slopes again two years after my injury, Paul demanded I buy one, too. And as Paul is a very safe bicyclist, nothing burns us up more than when we see people riding at top speed on a traffic-filled road with no helmet on—or worse, parents who make their kids wear helmets but don't model the behavior themselves. What, like the pavement is going to feel softer on your head because you're an adult? Nice example you're setting there, mom and dad.

I strongly believe that your brain function impacts your personality, but it doesn't have to define who you are. My cognitive deficits and emotional changes threatened to change my very core, leaving paralyzing fear, sadness and frustration in their wake. But the ability to fight through them, to keep trying to find a way around them, to deal with the tears by trying to find something to laugh at—that's all a very real part of who I was before the injury. These days, I realize that this desire to keep moving forward, to keep pushing through, is what makes me who I am—pre- or post-brain injury. As a result, the success or failure of the attempt doesn't really matter.

My hope is twofold. First, that people take brain injury more seriously and understand what its effects can be on those they know and love. And, second, that it doesn't take a brain aneurysm for people to learn the lessons I learned about slowing down, finding the humor, having more patience and savoring each activity in our 24/7 connected world.

Everyday challenges can present a new opportunity to reboot, start over and reframe the conversation with your work, your relationships—and with yourself. It's not easy and, like me, you won't be great at it every single day.

But again, it's the attempt that matters the most, not the outcome.

THE NEW ME

MY LIFE CONTINUES to ebb and flow, just like anyone else's. The reality of a near-death experience that people don't talk about is that you eventually get back on the hamster wheel like the rest of the world. I may have gotten my opportunity to "repack my suitcase" but, like any good spring cleaning, it tends to get cluttered up again. I wish I could say the philosophical musings of the last pages impact me each and every day, but tell that to the stupid guy in front of me in traffic yesterday who waited for the light to turn a different shade of green, which caused me to miss the left turn and then get stuck by the rising drawbridge when I was already late. My annoyed honking must not have seemed so Zen-like to him at that moment in time.

I am a changed person in many respects and not just because of the cognitive glitches I had to learn to work around. Because I can only handle so much at one time, I try to focus more on quality rather than quantity. When my overwhelm triggers either a complete paralysis of thought or one of my now-familiar mild panic attacks, I am able to ride them out a bit better. I can stop, turn off the noise, ask the other person to politely wait while I deal with one thing at a time, and then move on. At least now I'm good at recognizing the warning signs of spinning into chaos, and I've learned how to slow down the record and play it at my speed, rather than letting it play me. I also am much more aware of my hyperfocus issues, so I make sure I leave good chunks of breaks in my schedule and always make time to step away and eat lunch, ideally around noon.

Due to my memory issues, I don't remember faces and names as well as I used to. While I still have a savant-like ability to recall some obscure supporting actor's name from a 1989 film, I'm not so good when it comes to new people. Networking events are a little more challenging than they used to be. But you know what? When I meet people, I now tell them, "Sorry if I have to ask you again, but I'm not great with names." Yes, this is a new label for me that I am now okay with wearing. Faces don't stick in my head as well as they used to either, and I'm often second-guessing myself when meeting someone for coffee after only seeing them once or twice. I'd make a lousy eyewitness to a crime.

Notepads and sticky notes now dot almost every room in my house, and I carry a pen and paper in my purse wherever I go. I absolutely have to write things down or the details slip completely out of my mind. I'm getting a little bit better by using other crutches: Asking Paul to remind me to do something, or even asking friends to "remind me to tell you that story about Chicago after I order my latte or I'll forget." Or even repeating a task over and over out loud—often to a quizzical Eddie who thinks something wonderful is about to happen—so I don't forget it while en route between the kitchen upstairs and my office downstairs.

I was able to rev up my consulting business again to great success, and now I just work a little bit differently to stay on top of and provide great client work. I limit the number of clients I can effectively handle at any one time to ensure all those balls stay juggled in the air. Luckily, my creativity was not impacted negatively and, because I'm better about setting boundaries, staying focused on the present and leaving space in my schedule, I'm actually able to be a lot more innovative in many respects.

The brilliant Lumosity online games, so important in those early days, have rekindled my addiction to completing crosswords and brain games. This was a love affair I started at age six or seven, when I was an early reader. These games help keep my mind sharp and hopefully, continue to reestablish those connections in my head. I'm like a content old woman, lying in bed at night or sitting on a plane, working on my puzzles.

As for my other little tiny baby aneurysm, it's doing just fine. Despite my efforts at exercise, nutrition and stress-relief, my blood pressure continues to be high so the doctor put me on beta blocker pills. Besides keeping my blood pressure at a stable 120 over 80 by controlling the adrenaline in my body, it has the nice side effect of taking the edge off of my daily anxiety. That has helped with some of the random emotional meltdowns over meaningless trifles.

The greatest gift I received from this whole experience was the gift of community and love. From my parents, brothers, sisters-in-law and Paul's family, who checked up on me and showered us with love, worry and support. From my amazing girlfriends—women I admire and adore for their strength, beauty and knowing exactly what to do when crisis hits. They took care of Paul, organized communications, tweezed my wayward brows, ensured that scented hand cream was nearby at all times and, of course, forced me to experiment with lots of funky hats when my hair was shaved off. And the love and community I received from distant friends, relatives and colleagues who reached out with a note, email or phone call to rally my spirits.

But most importantly, the greatest gift I received was from my patient and faithful husband. Our young marriage was tested, and I feel that we passed with flying colors. On your wedding day, you repeat those vows of "for better or worse, in sickness and in health" but your face is flushed with love as you're surrounded by happy friends and family. Your hair is perfect, your clothes pressed, and everything is sweetness and light. You're not thinking of ventilators, walkers, shaved heads or full-time caregivers. My husband proved that he took those vows seriously. Not to say our marriage will never be tested again, but how often does one get a trial run like this?

Because of how strongly my tribe rallied around me, I learned that it's okay to count on others. I don't have to be superwoman and do it all myself, and this was a humbling and important step to take. Asking for help in order to move forward is not the same thing as asking for a handout. I can stop trying to be Little Miss Perfect, and people will still love me and accept me for who I am, flaws and all.

I'm not perfect by any stretch of the imagination. I haven't reached some Buddhist-like state where I don't get caught up in the stresses of everyday. Even if you have an experience like this, you're going to regress and go back to the everyday fire-fighting and drama. But when I find myself spinning out of control with that stress and worry, oftentimes I'll look at Paul while I'm ranting about deadlines, traffic or demanding clients and he'll just stare back at me, waiting. As he catches my eye, I trail off and realize how ridiculous it all sounds. I take a breath and say, "But it doesn't matter because I'm still here."

And he'll say, "That's right. You're still here." And then we move on.

My walks with Eddie each morning help keep me grounded as well. Dogs are amazing creatures. They live in a constant state of expectation and hope: Will she drop that cookie on the floor? Are you putting on your jacket so we can go to the dog park? Is that package you're opening full of treats for me? You clapped your hands! Does that mean you want to pet me? Eddie gets excited by everything because he lives in the moment. We're walking by the canal and I'm thinking "Oh, I've got to meet with this person today, and I've got to call that client and what I'm going to do about this, blah, blah, blah, blah..." Eddie yanks me back into the present moment—literally—straining on his leash to sniff the same damn bush he's sniffed every time we've walked past it. He teaches me that on those walks I need to be present, and I need to be there with him. And when I'm not, he pulls me over to the side and I get back in it right away.

I'd always suspected that we humans could learn a lot from dogs. If we'd just stop talking and running around long enough to get their message.

Friends often comment on the utter randomness of my injury. I was fit, healthy, active. I don't smoke, I drink responsibly, I don't do drugs—and I still got knocked down by surprise. You just never know. Life is not a Hollywood studio film: you can't predict the ending.

We are all much more vulnerable than we think, no matter how hard we try to be healthy or how much we think we are invincible. Life can change in a snap. For me, I had some warning signs leading up to the hemorrhage, but for others, it can be as simple as racing your car through a parking lot, or skidding out on your motorcycle, or a chance x-ray for sinus problems leading to the discovery of a grapefruit-sized tumor. You just never know.

First thing in the morning, I yank off my pajamas and throw on my dog-walking clothes. As I zip up my jeans, I look down to see a precise yet faint white line about one-and-a-half inches long to the right of my belly button. I rub my hand over it every day. The scar from the shunt placement surgery has healed with such precision, it's rather a work of art. Now it comforts me and reminds me of how truly strong I am, even when I feel weak.

I look in the mirror each night as I get ready for bed. In the inside corner of my left eyeball, a miniscule dash of a dark line stares back at me. It looks like an eyelash, but there is no blowing it away. A tiny incision scar from my retinal reattachment surgery almost always brings back the memory of searing pain from my two eye operations. But I'm grateful I can even see that scar.

I pull my hair back into a ponytail to tuck under my baseball cap. As I run my fingers through the right side of my hair, I feel a marked ridge about two inches long protruding slightly from my skull. It feels like the spine of a tiny brontosaurus or something, with all its bumps and nodules. I trace the thin tube trailing from it down behind my right ear, then across the front of my neck and follow it as it makes its way down the center of my chest before it then disappears into the depths of my abdomen. That small scar on my stomach marks the spot where, deep within me, a device exists to drain fluid that once threatened to crush my brain.

My fingers flutter to my chest where I trace the tube and I silently thank God for my husband, my family and my friends.

In a fit of poetic irony that my romantic side just can't ignore, I type the words of this last chapter on the third anniversary of the day I almost died: August 4, 2011. I'm nothing if not dramatic. Yes, I will probably remember this day for the rest of my life.

My name is Maria Ross. I almost died on August 4, 2008, but I'm still here. While not wise or profound or prolific, all I can say is, "Hurrah!" This seems appropriate.

This event forced me to look at my life differently, to reframe everything from my definition of success to my purpose in the world. I've learned what I can let slide and on what I should stay focused.

Your challenges may not be this traumatic (and I hope in some way I save you the trouble of taking this kind of extreme hit), but we can both ask ourselves the same questions as often as possible: "What really makes me me, and what gifts can I share? How will I use those gifts in the time I've been given, and how many lives can I touch?"

RESOURCES

Lumosity   www.lumosity.com

The website that helped me get my cognitive edge back can also help you with brain-training exercises that "can make you smarter and more mentally fit." Their games are developed using the latest information in neuroscience. They offer both free games and paid memberships.

Brain Injury Association of America (BIA)   www.biausa.org

From their website: "The Brain Injury Association of America (BIAA) is the voice of brain injury. We are dedicated to increasing access to quality health care and raising awareness and understanding of brain injury through advocacy, education and research. With a nationwide network of more than 40 chartered state affiliates and hundreds of local chapters and support groups, we provide help, hope and healing for individuals who live with brain injury, their families and the professionals who serve them."

Brain Injury Association of Washington (BIAWA)
www.braininurywa.org

This Washington state chapter of the BIA provides support, advocacy, education and preventive services. Their mission is "to increase public awareness, support, and hope for those affected by brain injury through education, assistance, and advocacy." They also operate a phone helpline specific to traumatic brain injury (TBI) that offers information, referrals, and over-the-phone and in-person resource management to thousands of brain injury survivors and their families. The BIAWA often partners with other organizations to help survivors of acquired brain injury (ABI) as well. This non-profit organization supports legislation to protect kids in school sports. In 2010, the BIAWA played a crucial role in passing Washington's Lystedt Law, named after an injured young football player. Now, twenty-two states have adopted this law, which requires young athletes who've suffered concussions to get medical clearance before competing again.

PubMed   www.ncbi.nlm.nih.gov/pubmed/

For medical studies, journal articles and any other current and medically sound information and science. From their website: "PubMed comprises more than 21 million citations for biomedical literature from MEDLINE, life science journals, and online books. Citations may include links to full-text content from PubMed Central and publisher web sites."

WebMD   www.webMD.com

For quick lookups and explanations about common health issues, "WebMD provides valuable health information, tools for managing your health, and support to those who seek information." I often consult this site when I don't understand terms in my medical reports or need information explained in layman's terms.

Rehab Without Walls   www.rehabwithoutwalls.com

This wonderful in-home therapy service helped me continue rehab and recovery after leaving the hospital. From their website: "Founded in 1991 as an alternative to traditional neurological rehabilitation programs, this unique service is delivered where patients need it most; in their own surroundings. Rehab Without Walls is focused on providing patients with the functional skills necessary to participate in practical daily activities at home, school, work or in the community where they live." They currently serve ten states, including Alaska, Arizona, California, Idaho, Michigan, Nevada, Oregon, Texas, Utah and Washington. If they do not serve your area, I'm sure there is a similar organization that does, so ask your doctor or healthcare provider.

CaringBridge   www.caringbridege.com

My friends created an online journal and guestbook on this website to keep others informed of my progress. From their website: "CaringBridge provides free websites that connect people experiencing a significant health challenge to family and friends, making each health journey easier. CaringBridge is powered by generous donors. CaringBridge websites offer a personal and private space to communicate and show support, saving time and emotional energy when health matters most. The websites are easy to create and use. Authors add health updates and photos to share their story while visitors leave messages of love, hope and compassion in the guestbook."

REBOOTING MY BRAIN . . . **207**

ACKNOWLEDGEMENTS

There are so many people to thank for helping me put this story out into the world.

To the dedicated doctors, nurses and staff of the University of Washington Medical Center and Harborview Medical Center for saving my life and comforting my family. Your caliber of care—and caring—is second to none. Special thanks to Dr. Basavaraj Ghodke, Dr. James Kinyoun, Dr. Mary Pepping, Dr. Michael Souter and Dr. Ivan Molton, who not only cared for me and helped in my recovery, but generously gave their time and resources to ensure I had my facts straight. To Carrel Sheldon, Hollis Ryan, Andrea Dotson, Debby Nagusky, Cindy Sayre and the rest of the dedicated Patient- and Family-Centered Care team and Patient and Family Education Committee at UWMC. Your work truly improves and touches lives. And to Tina Mankowski and Suzanne McCoy at UW Medicine for your time and support.

Thank you to my family for your love and support and for dropping everything to be with us. I am blessed to have you all, especially after such sadness that I saw. To Carrie, Becky, Elizabeth, Mary, John, Tracy, Ursula, Monty, Betsy, Warren, Barb and Guy for truly being there through the very worst times and never letting us lose hope. To Tim, Jill, Jeff, Kerry and Eliot, thank you for being there and opening your hearts (and homes) to us so early in our friendship. To Melody, Bridget and Judy, who cheered me on in the early days—and continue to do so. Thanks to friends far and wide who called, emailed, posted in my online journal, sent a card or contributed to our emergency fund. As Shakespeare said more eloquently than I ever could, "How far that little candle throws his beams! So shines a good deed in a weary world." Thank you for your light in our darkest times and for sharing our successes as well.

To all of my in-patient and out-patient therapists, many of whom I can't remember by name. If you dealt with me in the early days, sorry if I was an emotional brat! Thanks for helping me move forward. To every EMT, medical worker, nurse or doctor who played a role in my care: thank you for your efforts.

To the talented Kim Pearson for her keen developmental editing and objective eye. To Lori Zue for great feedback, brutal honesty and meticulous copyediting to help make my story the best it could be. To Robyn Fritz for getting me started. To Whitney Keyes for your constant cheerleading. To Ingrid Ricks and Wendy Hinman for your writing support and enthusiasm. To Juli Saeger Russell for the book cover and print layout and to eBook Architects for their e-book formatting. To Janica Smith for her admin assitance and support.

To Eddie the Wonder Dog, whose soulful eyes, wiggly butt and playful licks can heal any wound, visible or not. Thank you, my little buddy.

And to Paul. Words are not enough. You are my everything, and I literally would not be here if it weren't for you. Doesn't mean that gets you out of taking out the trash, but it does mean you have my heart forever.

ABOUT THE AUTHOR

Maria Ross is a consultant, writer, speaker and actress who believes that cash flow and creativity are not mutually exclusive. She writes frequently about branding, entrepreneurship, inspiration and even great wine, for such outlets as *San Francisco Downtown*, IntoWine.com, Sharp Skirts, DiningOutSF, Entrepreneur.com, American Express Open Forum and Seattle Business. Maria's first book, *Branding Basics for Small Business*, has been praised by marketing experts and best-selling authors alike. Maria is also a dynamic and sought-after speaker and has been featured in *Entrepreneur Magazine* and on MSNBC and KUOW Seattle. She is a lover of animals, red wine, travel, independent film, crime dramas, dry humor, football and *Jeopardy*. Maria lives in Seattle but is soon moving back to the San Francisco area with her husband Paul and their Black Lab mix, Eddie.

Follow Maria on Twitter (@redslice) on Facebook (www.facebook.com/redslice) or visit her website, www.red-slice.com. You can also sign up to hear about book signings and events, as well as see photos on the official book website, www.rebootingmybrain.com.

GROUP DISCUSSION QUESTIONS FOR REBOOTING MY BRAIN

1. The author reflects on her brain aneurysm as a "gift." How is this crisis a gift in her life? What did it teach her? Have you ever had a crisis that made you stronger or changed your thinking for the better? Do you see it as a gift? Why or why not?

2. Community, acceptance, patience and finding the humor in a bad situation are some of the key themes in this story. Can you find examples of where these lessons appear throughout the book? Did you find other themes?

3. What is the significance of the author's curly red hair? What does it represent to her? What are some personal attributes—physical or otherwise—that you feel impact your sense of self?

4. Eddie, the author's dog, pops up throughout the story. What is the dog's initial role in her life? How does he help her during her recovery? What role do you think companion animals play in a human's health and healing?

5. The author describes the "perfect storm" of stress, chaos and change at the beginning of the story. Have you ever had that much overwhelming activity going on in your life? Did your health suffer because of it? What do you do to keep your health and emotional well-being in balance amidst stress and change?

6. What did you learn about brain injury in the story? Did any of it surprise you? What has been your experience with brain injury, either yourself or with someone close to you?

7. The author describes moments of survivor's guilt when considering other brain injury patients who didn't fare as well mentally and physically as she did. Have you ever come out of a crisis relatively unscathed and felt guilty about those who did not? Do you think this is a normal reaction among those with trauma or chronic illnesses?

8. What do you think of the author's rant about "bucket lists"? Do you find them valuable and inspiring things, or do you see them as adding

to the pressure to "live our best lives"? Why or why not? Do you have
a bucket list? What types of things does it include?

9. The author questions whether our personalities are formed by our
   brain function or if our innate personalities inform how our brain
   works. What do you believe and why? Do you think people are born
   with certain traits that impact how they think and operate, or do people
   merely display personality traits that are a result of the way their brain
   is wired? What are the implications of your theory on criminals or
   those who are completely self-sacrificing? Do you think people can
   change?

ENDNOTES

1. Wikipedia.org, from cited published medical papers at
   http://en.wikipedia.org/wiki/Glasgow_Coma_Scale

2. The Mayo Clinic, http://www.mayoclinic.com/health/stroke/DS00150

3. Medline Plus, a service of the U.S. National Library of Medicine,
   "Subarachnoid Hemorrhage," http://www.nlm.nih.gov/medlineplus/ency/
   article/000701.htm

4. Wikipedia.org, from cited published medical papers at
   http://en.wikipedia.org/wiki/Subarachnoid_hemorrhage

5. Brain Aneurysm Resources, BrainAneurysm.com,
   http://www.brainaneurysm.com/aneurysm-treatment.html

6. Brain Injury Association of America,
   http://www.biausa.org/FAQRetrieve.aspx?ID=43913

7. Wikipedia.org, from cited published medical papers at
   http://en.wikipedia.org/wiki/Terson_syndrome

8. Harborview Medical Center, Patient and Family Education Document,
   Department of Neurology Surgery, Cerebral Artery Aneurysm, January,
   2006

9. The Mayo Clinic, http://www.mayoclinic.com/health/c-difficile/DS00736

10. Harborview Medical Center, Patient and Family Education Document,
    Department of Neurology Surgery, Cerebral Artery Aneurysm, January,
    2006

11. Medline Plus, a service of the U.S. National Library of Medicine,
    "Increased Intracranial Pressure,"
    http://www.nlm.nih.gov/medlineplus/ency/article/000793.htm

12. Harborview Medical Center, Patient and Family Education Document, Shunting, Neurosurgery, January, 2006

13. Medline Plus, a service of the U.S. National Library of Medicine, "Ventriculoperitoneal Shunting," http://www.nlm.nih.gov/medlineplus/ency/article/003019.htm

14. U.S. News & World Report, "America's Best Hospitals," 2009

15. University of Washington Medical Center, Patient and Family Education Document, Improving Symptom Management Following Subarachnoid Hemorrhage: Fatigue

16. Harborview Medical Center, Patient and Family Education Document, Acute Care for Patients with Brain Injury, Neurosurgery, January, 2006

17. Mary Pepping, PhD, University of Washington Medical Center, Group Psychotherapy Workbook, "Summary of Brain Areas and Deficits Following Damage," 2009

18. Mary Pepping, PhD, University of Washington Medical Center, Patient and Family Education Documents, Psychotherapy Rehab Binder, "Most Commonly Cited Cognitive Deficits After Brain Injury, as noted in a 20-year review of the literature," 2009

19. University of Washington Medical Center, Patient and Family Education Documents, Psychotherapy Rehab Binder, "Common Organically Based Changes in Personality," 2009, and "Common Emotional Reactions Following Brain Injury," 2009

20. National Conference of State Legislatures, Traumatic Brain Injury Legislation, updated August 2011, www.ncsl.org

CPSIA information can be obtained at www.ICGtesting.com
Printed in the USA
LVOW101803230113

316974LV00032B/1488/P